CASTOR OIL BIE

The Complete Castor Oil Companion.Transform Your Health and Beauty with Natural Remedies | includes recipes

Lisa Winsdow

SUMMARY

CASTOR OIL BIBLE...1

Introduction...7

Welcome to the Castor Oil Bible...7

The Natural Remedy Revolution 7

Why Castor Oil?..7

How to Use This Book 8

Chapter 1: Understanding Castor Oil 11

History and Origins...11

Ancient Uses of Castor Oil 11

Castor Oil in Modern Medicine....................................12

Composition and Properties 13

What Makes Castor Oil Unique?...................................13

The Chemistry of Castor Oil 14

Chapter 2: Health Benefits of Castor Oil 16

Digestive Health...16

Castor Oil for Constipation Relief................................16

Detoxifying the Liver with Castor Oil..........................17

Immune System Boost...18

Enhancing Immunity Naturally....................................18

Castor Oil for Anti-Inflammatory Support...................20

Pain Relief...21

Managing Arthritis and Joint Pain...............................21

Castor Oil for Muscle Soreness 22

Chapter 3: Castor Oil for Skin Care 24

Daily Skin Care Routine...24

Moisturizing and Hydrating the Skin...........................24

Healing Dry and Cracked Skin 25

Treating Skin Conditions 26

Acne and Blemish Control 26

Eczema and Psoriasis Relief 27

Anti-Aging Benefits 29

Reducing Wrinkles and Fine Lines...............................29

Promoting Skin Elasticity 30

Chapter 4: Castor Oil for Hair Care 32

Hair Growth and Thickness 32

    Stimulating Hair Follicles 32

    Preventing Hair Loss 33

Scalp Health..34

    Treating Dandruff and Dry Scalp 34

    Balancing Scalp Oils 36

Conditioning and Shine...37

    Deep Conditioning Treatments...37

    Restoring Hair Shine and Softness...38

Chapter 5: Castor Oil for Women's Health................................40

Menstrual Health...40

    Easing Menstrual Cramps...40

    Regulating Menstrual Cycles...41

Pregnancy and Postpartum Care 42

    Using Castor Oil During Pregnancy 42

    Postpartum Recovery with Castor Oil...................................43

Hormonal Balance 45

    Supporting Hormonal Health Naturally.................................45

Chapter 6: Castor Oil in Home Remedies..................................46

First Aid Applications 46

    Treating Minor Cuts and Burns 47

    Castor Oil for Insect Bites and Stings 47

Everyday Ailments..49

    Relieving Constipation 49

    Alleviating Cold and Flu Symptoms.......................................50

Detoxification 51

    Castor Oil Packs 51

    Full-Body Detox Methods 52

Chapter 7: DIY Castor Oil Beauty Recipes................................55

Skin Care Recipes 55

    DIY Face Masks and Scrubs 56

    DIY Face Mask Recipe: 56

    DIY Face Scrub Recipe: 57

Hair Care Recipes 58

    Castor Oil Shampoos and Conditioners................................58

    DIY Castor Oil Conditioner Recipe: 59

Hair Growth Serums...60

DIY Hair Strengthening Serum Recipe: 61

Body Care Recipes **62**

Bath Oils and Body Scrubs 62

Hand and Foot Treatments 64

Chapter 8: Safety and Precautions..............................**67**

Understanding Dosages **67**

Recommended Dosages for Adults and Children............67

Avoiding Overuse and Potential Side Effects.................68

Interactions and Contraindications **69**

Safe Use with Medications...69

Who Should Avoid Castor Oil...70

Purchasing and Storing Castor Oil **72**

Selecting High-Quality Castor Oil 72

Proper Storage Techniques..73

Chapter 9: Sourcing and Sustainability **75**

Ethical Sourcing...**75**

How Castor Oil is Produced..75

Identifying Ethical Suppliers..76

Environmental Impact **78**

The Environmental Benefits of Castor Oil 78

Reducing Your Ecological Footprint................................79

Homemade Castor Oil Production................................**81**

Making Castor Oil at Home 81

Ensuring Purity and Quality...83

Chapter 10: Testimonials and Case Studies **85**

Real-Life Success Stories **85**

Health Transformations with Castor Oil.........................85

Beauty Enhancements Through Natural Remedies........85

Expert Opinions **86**

Insights from Health and Wellness Experts 86

Medical Perspectives on Castor Oil Use 86

Your Journey with Castor Oil **87**

Tracking Your Progress 87

Sharing Your Story..87

Conclusion...**88**

Bringing It All Together **88**

    Integrating Castor Oil into Your Daily Life 88

    Long-Term Benefits and Continued Use 88

Resources and Further Reading..**89**

    Additional Books and Articles...89

    Helpful Websites and Blogs..89

Introduction

Welcome to the Castor Oil Bible

The Natural Remedy Revolution

Welcome to the Castor Oil Bible, your comprehensive guide to understanding and utilizing one of nature's most powerful remedies. Over the centuries, castor oil has earned a reputation as a versatile and effective natural solution for a myriad of health and beauty concerns. As more people seek alternatives to synthetic pharmaceuticals and chemical-laden beauty products, the demand for natural remedies has surged. This revolution in natural health is driven by a growing awareness of the potential side effects of conventional treatments and a desire for safer, more holistic approaches.

The natural remedy revolution is not just a trend; it's a fundamental shift towards embracing the wisdom of ancient practices combined with modern scientific insights. Castor oil, with its rich history and proven benefits, stands at the forefront of this movement. It offers a remarkable range of applications, from promoting digestive health and enhancing skin and hair care to providing relief from common ailments. In this book, we delve into the myriad ways castor oil can be used to improve your well-being, providing you with the knowledge to harness its full potential.

Why Castor Oil?

Why focus on castor oil? This simple yet powerful oil, derived from the seeds of the Ricinus communis plant, has been used for thousands of years for its therapeutic properties. Ancient civilizations, including the Egyptians, Greeks, and Romans, revered castor oil for its healing abilities. Today, modern research continues to uncover the science behind these ancient claims, confirming its efficacy in various medical and cosmetic applications.

Castor oil is unique due to its high concentration of ricinoleic acid, a fatty acid that gives the oil its remarkable anti-inflammatory, antimicrobial, and moisturizing properties. This makes it an invaluable resource for treating a wide range of conditions, from skin disorders and hair loss to digestive issues and arthritis pain. Furthermore, castor oil's natural composition means it is generally safe for most people to use, with minimal risk of side effects when applied correctly.

By choosing castor oil, you are opting for a natural remedy that is both effective and sustainable. It aligns with a holistic approach to health and beauty, emphasizing prevention, natural healing, and the use of gentle, non-toxic ingredients. This book will guide you through the various ways you can incorporate castor oil into your daily routine, empowering you to take control of your health and beauty naturally.

How to Use This Book

The Castor Oil Bible is designed to be your go-to resource for everything related to castor oil. Whether you are new to natural remedies or a seasoned enthusiast, this book provides valuable insights and practical advice to help you make the most of this incredible oil. Here's how to navigate through the chapters and make the most out of this guide:

1. **Understanding Castor Oil**: Start with Chapter 1 to gain a solid foundation of what castor oil is, its history, and its unique properties. This chapter sets

the stage for understanding why castor oil is so beneficial and how it works at a chemical level.

2. **Health Benefits of Castor Oil**: Move on to Chapter 2 to explore the various health benefits of castor oil. Learn about its role in digestive health, immune system support, and pain relief. This chapter includes detailed explanations and practical tips for using castor oil to enhance your overall health.

3. **Castor Oil for Skin Care**: Chapter 3 focuses on the cosmetic applications of castor oil, particularly for skin care. Discover how to incorporate castor oil into your daily skin care routine, and find solutions for common skin issues such as acne, eczema, and signs of aging.

4. **Castor Oil for Hair Care**: In Chapter 4, you will find everything you need to know about using castor oil to improve hair health. Learn about its benefits for hair growth, scalp health, and conditioning, with step-by-step guides for various hair treatments.

5. **Castor Oil for Women's Health**: Chapter 5 delves into the specific benefits of castor oil for women. Topics include menstrual health, pregnancy care, and hormonal balance, providing natural solutions for common female health concerns.

6. **Castor Oil in Home Remedies**: Chapter 6 expands on the practical uses of castor oil in everyday home remedies. From treating minor cuts and burns to relieving cold symptoms and promoting detoxification, this chapter offers a wealth of easy-to-follow remedies.

7. **DIY Castor Oil Beauty Recipes**: If you enjoy making your own beauty products, Chapter 7 is for you. Discover recipes for skin care, hair care, and

body care that you can create at home using castor oil and other natural ingredients.

8. **Safety and Precautions**: Chapter 8 is crucial for understanding the safe use of castor oil. Learn about recommended dosages, potential side effects, and interactions with other medications to ensure you use castor oil safely and effectively.

9. **Sourcing and Sustainability**: Chapter 9 covers the ethical and environmental aspects of castor oil production. Find out how to choose high-quality castor oil, support ethical suppliers, and even make your own castor oil at home.

10. **Testimonials and Case Studies**: Finally, Chapter 10 presents real-life success stories and expert opinions on the use of castor oil. Gain inspiration from others' experiences and learn how to track your progress and share your own journey with castor oil.

Each chapter is filled with detailed information, practical tips, and easy-to-follow instructions, making it easy to incorporate castor oil into your daily life. Whether you're looking to improve your health, enhance your beauty routine, or simply learn more about natural remedies, the Castor Oil Bible is your comprehensive guide to the wonders of castor oil. Welcome to a journey of natural healing and beauty—welcome to the Castor Oil Bible.

Chapter 1: Understanding Castor Oil

History and Origins

Castor oil, derived from the seeds of the Ricinus communis plant, has a storied history that spans thousands of years. Its origins trace back to ancient civilizations where it was esteemed for its remarkable healing properties. The earliest records of castor oil use date back to ancient Egypt around 4000 BC. The Egyptians referred to it as "Kiki oil" and used it extensively for medicinal and cosmetic purposes. It was found in Egyptian tombs, suggesting its high value and widespread use. Egyptians used castor oil as a laxative, to treat eye irritations, and as an important ingredient in their beauty regimens. Cleopatra is said to have used it to brighten the whites of her eyes. The oil's unique properties were so revered that it was considered a staple in many aspects of daily life.

Ancient Uses of Castor Oil

Beyond Egypt, castor oil's use spread to other ancient cultures. In ancient Greece and Rome, it was employed for similar medicinal and cosmetic purposes. The Greek physician Dioscorides documented its use as a powerful laxative in his medical texts, noting its ability to clear the bowels effectively. The Romans also recognized its value in treating skin conditions and maintaining overall health. Castor oil was a vital component of Ayurvedic medicine in India, where it was used to balance the body's doshas and treat various ailments, from arthritis to digestive disorders. Traditional Chinese medicine also utilized castor oil for its healing properties, particularly in treating inflammation and promoting digestive health. These ancient practices highlight the widespread acknowledgment of castor oil's efficacy across different cultures and time periods.

Castor Oil in Modern Medicine

As we transition to modern times, the medicinal use of castor oil has been scientifically validated and continues to evolve. In the 18th and 19th centuries, castor oil gained prominence in Europe and North America as a household remedy. It was commonly used as a laxative and for inducing labor in pregnant women. Despite advancements in synthetic medicines, castor oil has maintained its status in contemporary health practices due to its natural, holistic properties. Today, its applications have expanded far beyond its traditional uses. Modern medicine recognizes castor oil's anti-inflammatory and antimicrobial properties, making it useful in treating a variety of conditions. It is often recommended for skin ailments such as eczema, psoriasis, and acne, thanks to its ability to penetrate deep into the skin and provide lasting hydration and relief. Additionally, castor oil is used in the preparation of various pharmaceutical products, including coatings for pills and capsules due to its non-toxic nature.

In contemporary wellness circles, castor oil is celebrated for its versatility and effectiveness as a natural remedy. It is a staple in the world of naturopathy and holistic health, where it is used for detoxification and improving lymphatic circulation through castor oil packs. This traditional practice involves applying a cloth soaked in castor oil to the skin, usually on the abdomen, and is believed to enhance liver function and promote healing throughout the body. Moreover, research continues to explore and expand upon castor oil's potential benefits. Studies have shown promising results in its use for treating osteoarthritis, as an anti-inflammatory agent, and even in cancer therapy, highlighting its broad spectrum of applications.

By understanding the historical and modern uses of castor oil, we can appreciate its enduring significance and potential as a natural remedy. The journey of castor oil from ancient civilizations to modern medicine underscores its timeless value and the wisdom inherent in natural healing practices. This chapter lays the foundation for exploring the numerous ways in which castor oil can benefit our health and well-being in the chapters to come.

Composition and Properties

Castor oil's remarkable versatility and effectiveness can be attributed to its unique composition and properties. At its core, castor oil is a triglyceride, composed of fatty acids bound to glycerol. However, what sets it apart from other vegetable oils is its unusually high concentration of ricinoleic acid, which constitutes about 90% of its fatty acid content. This specific fatty acid is responsible for many of castor oil's therapeutic properties, including its potent anti-inflammatory, analgesic, and antimicrobial effects.

What Makes Castor Oil Unique?

The uniqueness of castor oil lies in its molecular structure, particularly the presence of ricinoleic acid. This monounsaturated, omega-9 fatty acid is rare in nature and gives castor oil its distinctive thick, viscous texture. Ricinoleic acid has a hydroxyl group on the 12th carbon atom, a feature that contributes to its high solubility in alcohol and makes it a powerful emulsifier. This unique property allows castor oil to be easily absorbed into the skin, providing deep hydration and delivering its therapeutic effects more efficiently than other oils.

Moreover, ricinoleic acid imparts castor oil with its exceptional anti-inflammatory and pain-relieving properties. Studies have shown that it can inhibit the growth of several bacterial species, making castor oil an effective antimicrobial agent. This is particularly beneficial for skin health, as it can help reduce acne-causing bacteria and other skin infections. Additionally, the high viscosity of castor oil forms a protective barrier on the skin, which helps retain moisture and promotes healing of dry, damaged skin.

Castor oil's unique composition also includes minor components such as linoleic acid (omega-6 fatty acid), oleic acid (omega-9 fatty acid), and stearic acid. These fatty acids complement the actions of ricinoleic acid, enhancing the oil's emollient properties and contributing to its overall effectiveness as a moisturizer and healing agent. The presence of these fatty acids also makes castor oil a versatile ingredient in cosmetic formulations, offering benefits such as improved skin elasticity and reduced appearance of fine lines and wrinkles.

The Chemistry of Castor Oil

Understanding the chemistry of castor oil provides further insight into why it is so effective in various applications. The molecular structure of ricinoleic acid, with its hydroxyl group, not only enhances the oil's solubility and absorption but also plays a crucial role in its pharmacological activities. This hydroxyl group is believed to be responsible for the oil's ability to modulate inflammatory pathways in the body, thus explaining its widespread use in treating inflammatory conditions.

In addition to its primary fatty acid content, castor oil contains several other bioactive compounds that contribute to its medicinal properties. These include tocopherols (vitamin E), which act as antioxidants, protecting the skin from oxidative stress and free radical damage. The presence of phytosterols in castor oil further enhances its anti-inflammatory and immune-boosting properties, making it a valuable addition to both skincare and therapeutic regimens.

The chemistry of castor oil also reveals its potential as a carrier oil in aromatherapy and pharmaceutical applications. Its ability to dissolve various compounds and deliver them through the skin makes it an excellent medium for transdermal therapies. For instance, when combined with essential oils, castor oil can enhance their penetration and effectiveness, making it a preferred choice for massage oils and topical treatments.

Furthermore, the unique chemical properties of castor oil extend to industrial applications. Its high hydroxyl value and viscosity make it an ideal raw material for producing lubricants, plastics, and synthetic resins. This versatility underscores the broad spectrum of castor oil's utility, from medicinal and cosmetic uses to industrial applications.

In summary, the distinctive composition and chemistry of castor oil, characterized by its high ricinoleic acid content and beneficial minor components, make it a powerful natural remedy with diverse applications. Its unique properties not only enhance its therapeutic effectiveness but also provide a scientific basis for its historical and modern uses. As we delve deeper into the various benefits and uses of castor oil in the following chapters, this foundational understanding will illuminate why castor oil remains a staple in natural health and wellness practices.

Chapter 2: Health Benefits of Castor Oil

Digestive Health

Castor oil has long been revered for its potent effects on digestive health, offering natural and effective solutions for common gastrointestinal issues. One of the primary benefits of castor oil in this domain is its ability to relieve constipation. This benefit, known and utilized for centuries, is attributed to the oil's unique composition and mechanism of action within the digestive tract.

Castor Oil for Constipation Relief

Constipation is a prevalent condition that affects people of all ages, causing discomfort and, in severe cases, leading to other health complications. Castor oil is an effective natural remedy for alleviating constipation due to its potent laxative properties. When ingested, castor oil is metabolized in the small intestine to ricinoleic acid, which then stimulates the intestinal muscles to contract. This action increases the movement of the intestines, helping to propel stool through the colon and promoting bowel movements.

The effectiveness of castor oil as a laxative has been well-documented in both historical texts and modern studies. Its rapid action makes it a go-to remedy for those seeking immediate relief from constipation. Typically, castor oil works within two to six hours of ingestion, making it a reliable option for those in need of quick results. It is important, however, to use castor oil with caution and in appropriate dosages to avoid potential side effects such as cramping or diarrhea.

To use castor oil for constipation relief, adults typically take a dose of about one to two tablespoons. It is often recommended to mix the oil with a juice or another flavored liquid to mask its strong taste. For children, the dosage is significantly lower and should be administered under the guidance of a healthcare professional. While castor oil is effective, it is not intended for long-term use. Chronic constipation should be addressed with a healthcare provider to identify and treat underlying causes.

Detoxifying the Liver with Castor Oil

Beyond its role in relieving constipation, castor oil is also celebrated for its detoxifying effects on the liver. The liver plays a crucial role in detoxifying the body, processing toxins, and maintaining overall health. A healthy liver is essential for the efficient functioning of various bodily systems, including digestion, metabolism, and immune response. Castor oil can support liver health and aid in its detoxification processes.

One of the traditional methods of using castor oil for liver detoxification is through the application of castor oil packs. This method involves soaking a piece of cloth in castor oil and placing it over the liver area, typically on the right side of the abdomen. The cloth is then covered with a plastic wrap and a hot water bottle or heating pad to enhance absorption and promote circulation. This practice is believed to stimulate the liver's detoxification processes, reduce inflammation, and improve lymphatic drainage.

Castor oil packs are often used as part of holistic detoxification programs. Regular use of castor oil packs can help reduce symptoms of liver congestion, such as bloating, fatigue, and digestive discomfort. The application of heat during the process not only facilitates the absorption of castor oil into the skin but also relaxes the muscles and improves blood flow, further supporting detoxification.

Scientific research supports the anti-inflammatory and detoxifying properties of castor oil, which can be beneficial for liver health. The high concentration of ricinoleic acid in castor oil contributes to its ability to reduce inflammation and support the liver's natural detoxification pathways. Additionally, the application of castor oil packs may stimulate the production of bile, a vital digestive fluid produced by the liver, aiding in the breakdown and elimination of fats and toxins.

Incorporating castor oil into a liver detox routine can be a natural and effective way to support liver function and overall health. However, it is important to approach detoxification practices mindfully and consult with a healthcare professional, especially for individuals with pre-existing health conditions or those taking medications.

In conclusion, castor oil offers significant benefits for digestive health, particularly in relieving constipation and supporting liver detoxification. Its unique properties and mechanisms of action make it a valuable natural remedy for promoting gastrointestinal well-being. As we explore further into the health benefits of castor oil, it becomes evident that this versatile oil holds a prominent place in natural health and wellness practices.

Immune System Boost

Enhancing Immunity Naturally

Castor oil is not only beneficial for digestive health but also plays a significant role in enhancing the body's immune system. The immune system is our first line of defense against infections and diseases, and maintaining its optimal function is crucial for overall health. Castor oil's unique properties can boost immune function naturally, offering a non-toxic, holistic approach to supporting immune health.

One of the ways castor oil enhances immunity is through its ability to improve lymphatic drainage. The lymphatic system is an essential part of the immune system, responsible for transporting lymph, a fluid containing white blood cells, throughout the body. This system helps remove toxins, waste, and other unwanted materials from the body. Poor lymphatic circulation can lead to a buildup of toxins and a weakened immune response. Castor oil can help improve lymphatic flow, thereby enhancing the body's ability to fight off infections and maintain homeostasis.

Topical application of castor oil packs, a traditional method, is particularly effective in stimulating the lymphatic system. When applied to the skin, especially over lymph nodes or the abdomen, castor oil is absorbed and can increase the movement of lymph fluid. This practice supports detoxification and can help reduce symptoms of lymphatic congestion, such as swelling, inflammation, and fatigue. Regular use of castor oil packs can thus contribute to a more robust immune system and better overall health.

In addition to improving lymphatic circulation, castor oil also has direct antimicrobial properties that can help defend the body against harmful pathogens. The high ricinoleic acid content in castor oil is known for its ability to inhibit the growth of bacteria, viruses, and fungi. This makes castor oil a valuable natural remedy for preventing and treating infections, further supporting the immune system.

Castor Oil for Anti-Inflammatory Support

Another critical aspect of immune health is the body's ability to manage inflammation. While acute inflammation is a natural and necessary response to injury or infection, chronic inflammation can weaken the immune system and lead to various health issues, including autoimmune diseases, cardiovascular problems, and cancer. Castor oil's potent anti-inflammatory properties make it an excellent natural remedy for managing inflammation and supporting immune health.

Ricinoleic acid, the primary fatty acid in castor oil, has been shown to exert significant anti-inflammatory effects. When applied to the skin, it can penetrate deep into the tissues and reduce inflammation at the cellular level. This is particularly beneficial for conditions such as arthritis, where chronic inflammation leads to joint pain and stiffness. By reducing inflammation, castor oil not only alleviates pain but also prevents further tissue damage and supports the healing process.

Moreover, the anti-inflammatory effects of castor oil are not limited to topical application. When taken internally, castor oil can help reduce inflammation in the digestive tract and other internal organs. This is beneficial for conditions like inflammatory bowel disease (IBD), where chronic inflammation affects the lining of the intestines. By soothing the inflamed tissues, castor oil can help manage symptoms and promote intestinal health.

Castor oil's anti-inflammatory properties also extend to its ability to modulate the immune response. In autoimmune conditions, where the immune system mistakenly attacks the body's own tissues, reducing inflammation can help regulate immune activity and prevent flare-ups. This makes castor oil a valuable addition to the management of autoimmune diseases, offering a natural way to balance immune function and reduce reliance on pharmaceutical anti-inflammatories.

In summary, castor oil provides multiple benefits for boosting the immune system naturally. Its ability to enhance lymphatic drainage, provide antimicrobial protection, and reduce inflammation makes it a powerful ally in maintaining immune health. By incorporating castor oil into your wellness routine, you can support your body's natural defenses and promote overall health. As we continue to explore the health benefits of castor oil, its role in enhancing immunity and providing anti-inflammatory support becomes increasingly evident, underscoring its value in natural health practices.

Pain Relief

Managing Arthritis and Joint Pain

Arthritis and joint pain are common ailments that affect millions of people worldwide, often leading to decreased mobility and quality of life. Castor oil has been recognized for its ability to provide natural relief from these conditions. Its potent anti-inflammatory and analgesic properties make it an effective remedy for managing arthritis and alleviating joint pain.

The high concentration of ricinoleic acid in castor oil plays a crucial role in its pain-relieving capabilities. When applied topically, castor oil penetrates deeply into the skin and underlying tissues, reducing inflammation and swelling in the affected joints. This action helps to alleviate pain and improve joint mobility. The use of castor oil for arthritis has been supported by both historical anecdotes and modern scientific studies, which highlight its effectiveness in reducing pain and inflammation.

To use castor oil for arthritis and joint pain, one can apply it directly to the affected area, massaging it in gently to ensure deep penetration. For enhanced results, a castor oil pack can be used. This involves soaking a piece of flannel cloth in castor oil, placing it over the painful joint, covering it with plastic wrap, and applying heat with a heating pad. This method not only helps to soothe pain and inflammation but also improves circulation in the area, promoting healing and relief.

Castor oil's effectiveness in managing arthritis and joint pain makes it a valuable addition to natural pain management strategies. It offers a safe and non-invasive alternative to conventional pain medications, which often come with significant side effects. By incorporating castor oil into a regular pain management routine, individuals can experience long-term relief and improved joint health.

Castor Oil for Muscle Soreness

In addition to its benefits for arthritis and joint pain, castor oil is also highly effective in relieving muscle soreness. Muscle soreness can result from a variety of causes, including intense physical activity, injury, or chronic conditions such as fibromyalgia. Castor oil's natural analgesic and anti-inflammatory properties make it an excellent remedy for easing muscle discomfort and promoting recovery.

The application of castor oil to sore muscles helps to reduce inflammation and improve blood flow to the affected area. This increased circulation helps to remove toxins and metabolic waste products that accumulate in the muscles during strenuous activity, thereby reducing soreness and promoting faster recovery. The warming sensation of castor oil also provides immediate relief by relaxing tense muscles and reducing spasms.

To use castor oil for muscle soreness, simply massage the oil into the sore muscles, focusing on areas of tension and discomfort. The oil's thick consistency and deep-penetrating properties ensure that it reaches the underlying tissues, providing effective relief. For even greater benefits, castor oil can be combined with other essential oils known for their muscle-relaxing properties, such as peppermint or eucalyptus oil. This combination enhances the overall therapeutic effect, providing a soothing and invigorating experience.

Castor oil packs can also be used for muscle soreness, similar to the method used for joint pain. By applying a castor oil-soaked cloth to the sore muscles and using heat, one can achieve deeper penetration and more significant relief. This method is particularly beneficial for larger muscle groups, such as the back or thighs, where extensive soreness may be present.

The regular use of castor oil for muscle soreness not only provides immediate relief but also helps to prevent future discomfort. By keeping muscles supple and well-nourished, castor oil supports overall muscle health and resilience, making it an essential tool for athletes and individuals with physically demanding lifestyles.

In conclusion, castor oil offers a powerful, natural solution for pain relief, effectively managing arthritis, joint pain, and muscle soreness. Its unique composition and properties make it a versatile remedy that addresses the root causes of pain and inflammation, providing both immediate and long-term benefits. As we explore the various applications of castor oil in pain management, its role as a holistic and effective natural remedy becomes increasingly clear, highlighting its importance in maintaining overall health and well-being.

Chapter 3: Castor Oil for Skin Care

Daily Skin Care Routine

Castor oil has long been esteemed for its profound benefits in skin care, offering a natural solution to various skin conditions and enhancing the overall health and appearance of the skin. Incorporating castor oil into your daily skin care routine can provide substantial benefits, ensuring your skin remains moisturized, hydrated, and protected from environmental damage. Its unique composition, rich in ricinoleic acid, along with its high content of fatty acids, makes it an excellent choice for daily use.

A well-rounded skin care routine with castor oil can start with cleansing. Castor oil acts as a gentle and effective cleanser, suitable for removing dirt, makeup, and impurities from the skin without stripping it of its natural oils. To use castor oil as a cleanser, apply a small amount to your fingertips and massage it into your skin in circular motions. This method, often referred to as the oil cleansing method, dissolves impurities and unclogs pores, leaving the skin clean and soft. Follow this by wiping away the oil with a warm, damp cloth to remove excess oil and debris, revealing a refreshed complexion.

Moisturizing and Hydrating the Skin

One of the standout properties of castor oil is its exceptional ability to moisturize and hydrate the skin. The high concentration of fatty acids in castor oil penetrates deeply into the skin, providing long-lasting hydration and creating a barrier that locks in moisture. This makes it an ideal moisturizer for all skin types, particularly for those with dry or sensitive skin.

To use castor oil as a moisturizer, apply a few drops to your face and neck after cleansing. Gently massage the oil into the skin, allowing it to absorb fully. The thick, emollient nature of castor oil ensures that even a small amount can provide ample hydration, making it a cost-effective addition to your skincare routine. For those with oily or acne-prone skin, blending castor oil with lighter oils, such as jojoba or grapeseed oil, can balance the skin's oil production and prevent clogged pores.

In addition to facial use, castor oil can be applied to the body to hydrate dry areas such as elbows, knees, and feet. Regular application can help maintain smooth, supple skin, preventing dryness and flakiness. Its ability to penetrate deeply into the skin makes it particularly effective for keeping the skin hydrated and protected from harsh environmental factors, such as cold weather and dry air.

Healing Dry and Cracked Skin

Castor oil is also renowned for its healing properties, making it an excellent remedy for dry and cracked skin. The rich, thick consistency of castor oil provides a protective barrier that not only hydrates but also heals damaged skin. Its anti-inflammatory and antimicrobial properties further aid in soothing irritated skin and preventing infections.

For treating dry and cracked skin, especially on the hands and feet, apply a generous amount of castor oil to the affected areas before bedtime. Covering the area with cotton gloves or socks helps to enhance absorption and prevent the oil from transferring to bed linens. By morning, the skin is typically softer and more hydrated, with visible improvement in texture and reduced cracks.

Castor oil can also be used to treat more severe skin conditions, such as eczema and psoriasis. Its anti-inflammatory properties help to reduce redness, swelling, and itching associated with these conditions, while its moisturizing effects alleviate dryness and flaking. Applying castor oil regularly to affected areas can significantly improve the condition of the skin, promoting healing and comfort.

Incorporating castor oil into your daily skin care routine can transform the health and appearance of your skin. Its moisturizing, hydrating, and healing properties make it a versatile and effective natural remedy for a wide range of skin concerns. As we delve deeper into the specific benefits and applications of castor oil for skin care in this chapter, you will discover how this remarkable oil can enhance your skin's beauty and health, providing a natural glow and resilience against daily stressors.

Treating Skin Conditions

Acne and Blemish Control

Acne and blemishes are common skin conditions that affect individuals of all ages, often causing physical discomfort and emotional distress. Castor oil, with its unique properties, offers a natural and effective solution for managing acne and controlling blemishes. The key to castor oil's effectiveness in acne treatment lies in its high content of ricinoleic acid, which has potent anti-inflammatory and antibacterial properties.

When applied to the skin, castor oil penetrates deeply into the pores, dissolving excess sebum, dirt, and dead skin cells that can clog pores and lead to acne breakouts. Its antibacterial properties help to reduce the presence of acne-causing bacteria, such as Propionibacterium acnes, thereby preventing and treating infections. Additionally, the anti-inflammatory properties of ricinoleic acid help to reduce redness, swelling, and irritation associated with acne.

To use castor oil for acne treatment, start by cleansing your face thoroughly. Apply a small amount of castor oil to the affected areas using a clean cotton swab or your fingertips, gently massaging it into the skin. For best results, leave the oil on overnight and rinse it off in the morning. This allows the oil to work effectively while you sleep, reducing inflammation and promoting healing. For those with oily or combination skin, mixing castor oil with lighter oils, such as jojoba or argan oil, can help balance oil production and prevent pore congestion.

Regular use of castor oil can help to control acne and prevent future breakouts. Its moisturizing properties also ensure that the skin remains hydrated and healthy, which is essential for maintaining a clear complexion. By incorporating castor oil into your skincare routine, you can achieve a natural, effective approach to managing acne and blemishes without the harsh side effects often associated with conventional treatments.

Eczema and Psoriasis Relief

Eczema and psoriasis are chronic inflammatory skin conditions characterized by dry, itchy, and inflamed patches of skin. These conditions can be particularly challenging to manage, often requiring long-term treatment and care. Castor oil, known for its soothing and healing properties, offers significant relief for individuals suffering from eczema and psoriasis.

The emollient properties of castor oil provide deep hydration, helping to restore the skin's natural moisture barrier and prevent further dryness and irritation. Its anti-inflammatory effects help to calm inflamed skin, reducing redness, itching, and discomfort. Moreover, the oil's ability to penetrate deeply into the skin ensures that it delivers these benefits effectively, promoting healing from within.

For treating eczema and psoriasis, apply a generous amount of castor oil to the affected areas, gently massaging it into the skin. For enhanced absorption and relief, consider using castor oil packs. Soak a piece of flannel cloth in castor oil, place it over the affected area, cover it with plastic wrap, and apply heat with a heating pad. This method not only enhances the oil's absorption but also provides soothing warmth, further reducing inflammation and discomfort.

In addition to its moisturizing and anti-inflammatory properties, castor oil has antimicrobial effects that help prevent infections in broken or damaged skin, a common concern in eczema and psoriasis. Regular application of castor oil can significantly improve the condition of the skin, alleviating symptoms and promoting overall skin health.

Castor oil can also be used as part of a broader skincare regimen for eczema and psoriasis. Combining it with other natural ingredients known for their soothing properties, such as aloe vera, chamomile, or calendula, can enhance its effectiveness. These combinations can provide a comprehensive approach to managing these chronic conditions, ensuring the skin remains hydrated, protected, and comfortable.

In summary, castor oil offers a natural, effective solution for treating various skin conditions, including acne, eczema, and psoriasis. Its unique properties, including its ability to deeply moisturize, reduce inflammation, and combat bacteria, make it a versatile and powerful tool in skincare. By incorporating castor oil into your daily routine, you can achieve significant improvements in your skin's health and appearance, providing relief from chronic conditions and promoting a clear, healthy complexion. As we continue to explore the benefits of castor oil for skin care, its role in treating and managing skin conditions becomes increasingly evident, highlighting its importance in natural skincare practices.

Anti-Aging Benefits

Reducing Wrinkles and Fine Lines

As we age, our skin naturally loses its elasticity and moisture, leading to the formation of wrinkles and fine lines. Castor oil, with its rich composition of fatty acids and potent antioxidants, offers a natural and effective solution for combating these signs of aging. One of the primary reasons castor oil is so beneficial in reducing wrinkles and fine lines is its ability to deeply penetrate the skin, delivering hydration and essential nutrients to the underlying tissues.

The high concentration of ricinoleic acid in castor oil helps to moisturize the skin, maintaining its softness and suppleness. This fatty acid, along with other beneficial components in the oil, forms a protective barrier on the skin, preventing moisture loss and keeping the skin hydrated for longer periods. Hydrated skin is less prone to developing wrinkles, as it remains plump and resilient.

Moreover, castor oil is rich in antioxidants, which play a crucial role in protecting the skin from damage caused by free radicals. Free radicals are unstable molecules that can damage collagen and elastin, the proteins responsible for maintaining the skin's structure and elasticity. By neutralizing these free radicals, the antioxidants in castor oil help to prevent and reduce the appearance of wrinkles and fine lines.

To incorporate castor oil into your anti-aging skincare routine, apply a small amount of oil to your face and neck after cleansing. Gently massage the oil into the skin, focusing on areas prone to wrinkles, such as around the eyes, mouth, and forehead. For enhanced benefits, castor oil can be combined with other anti-aging ingredients, such as rosehip oil or vitamin E, which further boost its effectiveness in reducing wrinkles and fine lines.

Regular use of castor oil can lead to noticeable improvements in the texture and appearance of the skin, providing a natural and effective way to combat the signs of aging.

Promoting Skin Elasticity

In addition to reducing wrinkles and fine lines, castor oil is highly effective in promoting skin elasticity. Elasticity is the skin's ability to return to its original shape after stretching or contracting, and it is a key factor in maintaining a youthful appearance. As we age, the production of collagen and elastin decreases, leading to a loss of elasticity and the formation of sagging skin.

Castor oil stimulates the production of collagen and elastin, enhancing the skin's structural integrity and elasticity. The fatty acids in castor oil penetrate deeply into the skin, nourishing the cells and promoting the synthesis of these vital proteins. This results in firmer, more resilient skin that is better able to withstand the effects of aging.

To promote skin elasticity with castor oil, apply it regularly to the face, neck, and other areas prone to sagging, such as the décolletage and hands. The oil's thick consistency ensures that it stays on the skin longer, allowing for maximum absorption and effectiveness. Massaging the oil into the skin in circular motions can also stimulate blood flow and enhance its benefits.

Incorporating castor oil into a comprehensive skincare routine can provide lasting improvements in skin elasticity. Combining it with other natural ingredients known for their anti-aging properties, such as hyaluronic acid, peptides, or aloe vera, can create a synergistic effect that enhances the overall health and appearance of the skin.

Moreover, castor oil's moisturizing properties help to maintain the skin's moisture balance, preventing dryness and flakiness, which can contribute to a loss of elasticity. Well-hydrated skin remains more pliable and resilient, reducing the likelihood of sagging and maintaining a youthful, radiant appearance.

In conclusion, castor oil offers significant anti-aging benefits, including the reduction of wrinkles and fine lines and the promotion of skin elasticity. Its unique composition of fatty acids and antioxidants makes it a powerful tool in natural skincare, providing a safe and effective alternative to synthetic anti-aging products. By incorporating castor oil into your daily skincare routine, you can achieve a more youthful, vibrant complexion, enhancing both the appearance and health of your skin. As we continue to explore the benefits of castor oil for skin care, its role in anti-aging becomes increasingly evident, underscoring its value in maintaining youthful, healthy skin.

Chapter 4: Castor Oil for Hair Care

Hair Growth and Thickness

Castor oil has garnered a well-deserved reputation as a potent natural remedy for enhancing hair growth and improving hair thickness. This versatile oil is packed with nutrients and fatty acids that nourish the scalp and hair follicles, promoting healthy hair growth and adding volume and strength to the hair. Its unique properties make it an invaluable addition to hair care routines for those seeking to combat thinning hair and stimulate robust hair growth.

The secret to castor oil's effectiveness in promoting hair growth lies in its high concentration of ricinoleic acid. This fatty acid has potent anti-inflammatory and antimicrobial properties that help maintain a healthy scalp environment, which is crucial for optimal hair growth. By reducing scalp inflammation and combating fungal and bacterial infections, castor oil creates a conducive environment for hair follicles to thrive.

Moreover, castor oil is rich in omega-6 and omega-9 fatty acids, which provide essential nourishment to the hair follicles. These fatty acids help to strengthen the hair shaft, reducing breakage and split ends. This results in thicker, healthier hair that is less prone to damage. Additionally, the oil's emollient properties ensure that the hair remains moisturized, preventing dryness and brittleness.

Stimulating Hair Follicles

Stimulating the hair follicles is key to promoting hair growth, and castor oil excels in this aspect. When massaged into the scalp, castor oil improves blood circulation, ensuring that the hair follicles receive an adequate supply of nutrients and oxygen.

This increased blood flow helps to revitalize dormant hair follicles and encourages the growth of new hair.

To stimulate hair follicles with castor oil, it is essential to use a regular scalp massage technique. Apply a small amount of castor oil to your fingertips and massage it into the scalp using circular motions. This not only helps the oil to penetrate deeply into the scalp but also boosts circulation and relaxes the scalp muscles. For best results, perform this massage for at least five to ten minutes before washing the hair. Doing this regularly can lead to significant improvements in hair growth and density.

Castor oil can also be combined with other natural ingredients known for their hair growth-stimulating properties. For example, mixing castor oil with essential oils such as peppermint or rosemary oil can enhance its effectiveness. These essential oils have been shown to stimulate blood flow to the scalp and promote hair growth. Adding a few drops of these oils to castor oil and massaging the mixture into the scalp can provide a synergistic effect, leading to even better results.

Preventing Hair Loss

Hair loss can be a distressing condition, but castor oil offers a natural solution to help prevent it. The nourishing and strengthening properties of castor oil make it an excellent remedy for combating hair loss and promoting the retention of healthy hair. By maintaining a healthy scalp and providing essential nutrients to the hair follicles, castor oil helps to prevent hair from falling out prematurely.

One of the primary causes of hair loss is the weakening of hair follicles, which can be exacerbated by factors such as stress, hormonal imbalances, and poor scalp health. Castor oil's ability to penetrate deeply into the scalp and strengthen the hair follicles makes it particularly effective in preventing hair loss. Its antifungal and antibacterial properties also help to keep the scalp healthy, reducing the risk of infections that can lead to hair loss.

For individuals experiencing hair loss, incorporating castor oil into their hair care routine can make a significant difference. Apply castor oil to the scalp and hair, focusing on areas where hair loss is most prominent. Leave the oil on for at least an hour before washing it out with a gentle shampoo. For intensive treatment, the oil can be left on overnight and rinsed out in the morning. Regular use of castor oil in this manner can help to reduce hair loss and promote the growth of strong, healthy hair.

In conclusion, castor oil is a powerful natural remedy for enhancing hair growth, stimulating hair follicles, and preventing hair loss. Its rich composition of nutrients and fatty acids, combined with its anti-inflammatory and antimicrobial properties, makes it an effective and versatile solution for various hair care needs. By incorporating castor oil into your hair care routine, you can achieve thicker, healthier hair and address common hair concerns naturally and effectively. As we continue to explore the benefits of castor oil for hair care, its role in promoting hair growth and preventing hair loss becomes increasingly evident, highlighting its importance in natural hair care practices.

Scalp Health

Treating Dandruff and Dry Scalp

Maintaining a healthy scalp is fundamental to achieving healthy hair, and castor oil excels in addressing common scalp issues such as dandruff and dry scalp. Dandruff, characterized by flaky and itchy scalp, can be both uncomfortable and embarrassing. Dry scalp, on the other hand, often leads to itching, irritation, and increased hair breakage. Castor oil's unique properties make it an excellent remedy for these conditions, offering soothing relief and promoting overall scalp health.

Dandruff is often caused by an overgrowth of a yeast-like fungus called Malassezia, which thrives on the scalp's natural oils. Castor oil's antifungal properties effectively combat this fungus, reducing the presence of dandruff. Additionally, its anti-inflammatory effects help to soothe an irritated scalp, reducing redness and itching associated with dandruff.

To treat dandruff with castor oil, mix it with a few drops of tea tree oil, known for its potent antifungal and antibacterial properties. Apply the mixture to the scalp and massage it in gently. Leave it on for at least 30 minutes before rinsing it out with a gentle shampoo. Regular application of this treatment can significantly reduce dandruff and prevent its recurrence, leading to a healthier, flake-free scalp.

For a dry scalp, castor oil provides deep hydration and nourishment. Its thick, viscous nature allows it to form a protective barrier on the scalp, locking in moisture and preventing further dryness. The high concentration of fatty acids in castor oil, particularly ricinoleic acid, penetrates deeply into the scalp, providing lasting hydration and relief from dryness.

To use castor oil for a dry scalp, warm a small amount of the oil and apply it directly to the scalp, massaging it in thoroughly. For best results, leave the oil on overnight, allowing it to penetrate and moisturize the scalp deeply. Cover your hair with a shower cap or a towel to prevent staining your bedding. In the morning, wash your hair with a mild shampoo. Regular use of castor oil in this manner will keep your scalp hydrated, reduce dryness, and promote a healthier scalp environment.

Balancing Scalp Oils

A well-balanced scalp oil level is essential for maintaining healthy hair and scalp. Both excessive oil production and insufficient oil production can lead to various scalp issues, including oily hair, dandruff, and dry scalp. Castor oil helps to regulate and balance the scalp's natural oil production, ensuring an optimal environment for hair growth.

For those with an oily scalp, castor oil can help to balance the production of sebum, the scalp's natural oil. Overactive sebaceous glands can lead to an oily scalp and hair, making it prone to dandruff and other scalp issues. Castor oil's astringent properties help to cleanse the scalp of excess oil and impurities, reducing the overproduction of sebum.

To balance an oily scalp, mix castor oil with lighter oils such as jojoba or grapeseed oil, which closely mimic the scalp's natural sebum. Apply the mixture to the scalp and massage it in gently. Leave it on for about 30 minutes before rinsing it out with a gentle, sulfate-free shampoo. This treatment helps to cleanse the scalp and regulate oil production, preventing the scalp from becoming too oily.

Conversely, for those with a dry scalp, castor oil can provide the necessary moisture to balance oil levels. Its emollient properties ensure that the scalp remains hydrated, preventing dryness and flakiness. Regular application of castor oil can help to maintain the scalp's natural moisture balance, promoting a healthy environment for hair growth.

Balancing scalp oils is also crucial for preventing hair loss and promoting hair health. A well-moisturized scalp reduces the risk of hair breakage and promotes stronger, healthier hair. By keeping the scalp's oil levels balanced, castor oil helps to maintain overall scalp health and supports the growth of thick, healthy hair.

In conclusion, castor oil is a versatile and effective remedy for maintaining scalp health. Its ability to treat dandruff, hydrate a dry scalp, and balance scalp oils makes it an invaluable addition to any hair care routine. By incorporating castor oil into your scalp care regimen, you can address common scalp issues naturally and effectively, promoting a healthy scalp and beautiful, resilient hair. As we delve deeper into the benefits of castor oil for hair care, its role in maintaining scalp health becomes increasingly clear, underscoring its importance in natural hair care practices.

Conditioning and Shine

Deep Conditioning Treatments

Castor oil is renowned for its deep conditioning properties, making it an excellent natural treatment for restoring moisture and vitality to the hair. Its thick, viscous texture allows it to penetrate deeply into the hair shaft, delivering essential nutrients and hydration. This deep conditioning capability is particularly beneficial for dry, damaged, or chemically-treated hair, which often requires intensive moisture to regain its health and strength.

Deep conditioning treatments with castor oil can transform the hair by infusing it with moisture and nutrients. To create an effective deep conditioning treatment, combine castor oil with other nourishing ingredients like coconut oil, honey, or avocado. These natural ingredients work synergistically to enhance the conditioning effects of castor oil, providing comprehensive nourishment to the hair.

To perform a deep conditioning treatment, start by applying the castor oil mixture to clean, damp hair. Section your hair to ensure even application, and massage the oil mixture from the roots to the ends, focusing on the most damaged areas. Once the oil is evenly distributed, cover your hair with a shower cap or a warm towel. The heat helps to open the hair cuticles, allowing the oil to penetrate more deeply. Leave the treatment on for at least 30 minutes, or for an intensive treatment, leave it on overnight. After the treatment, rinse your hair thoroughly with a gentle shampoo to remove the excess oil.

Regular deep conditioning treatments with castor oil can significantly improve the texture and health of your hair. They help to repair damage, reduce breakage, and promote overall hair resilience. The result is deeply conditioned, nourished hair that is soft, smooth, and full of life.

Restoring Hair Shine and Softness

In addition to its deep conditioning benefits, castor oil is highly effective in restoring shine and softness to the hair. Dull, lifeless hair can be a result of various factors, including environmental damage, heat styling, and the use of harsh hair products. Castor oil's rich composition of fatty acids and vitamins provides the nourishment needed to revive and rejuvenate the hair, enhancing its natural shine and softness.

Castor oil smoothens the hair cuticle, which is the outermost layer of the hair. A smooth cuticle reflects light better, giving the hair a healthy, glossy appearance. The emollient properties of castor oil also help to seal in moisture, preventing dryness and frizz. This makes the hair feel softer and more manageable.

To restore shine and softness, apply a small amount of castor oil to your hair as a leave-in treatment. For best results, use the oil sparingly to avoid weighing down your hair. Start by rubbing a few drops of castor oil between your palms to warm it up, then run your hands through your hair, focusing on the mid-lengths and ends.

This helps to distribute the oil evenly and ensures that it coats the hair strands, providing a protective and moisturizing barrier.

For an extra boost of shine, you can also use castor oil as a finishing oil after styling. Apply a small amount to your fingertips and lightly run them over the surface of your hair. This helps to tame flyaways, reduce frizz, and add a polished finish to your hairstyle.

Combining castor oil with other shine-enhancing ingredients, such as argan oil or jojoba oil, can further amplify its benefits. These lightweight oils blend well with castor oil and enhance its ability to smooth the hair cuticle and add shine. Mixing a few drops of these oils with castor oil creates a powerful, natural shine serum that can be used regularly to maintain glossy, soft hair.

In conclusion, castor oil is a versatile and effective solution for conditioning and enhancing the shine and softness of your hair. Its deep conditioning treatments repair and nourish the hair, while its ability to restore shine and softness revives dull, damaged hair. By incorporating castor oil into your hair care routine, you can achieve healthy, radiant hair that looks and feels its best. As we continue to explore the benefits of castor oil for hair care, its role in conditioning and adding shine becomes increasingly evident, highlighting its importance in natural hair care practices.

Chapter 5: Castor Oil for Women's Health

Menstrual Health

Castor oil has long been valued for its medicinal properties, and its benefits extend significantly to various aspects of women's health. One of the key areas where castor oil proves exceptionally beneficial is in managing menstrual health. Menstrual issues such as cramps and irregular cycles are common concerns for many women, often leading to discomfort and stress. Castor oil offers natural, effective solutions for easing menstrual cramps and regulating menstrual cycles, providing relief and promoting overall reproductive health.

Easing Menstrual Cramps

Menstrual cramps, or dysmenorrhea, can be debilitating for many women, causing significant pain and discomfort during their menstrual periods. The anti-inflammatory and analgesic properties of castor oil make it an excellent natural remedy for alleviating these cramps. The high concentration of ricinoleic acid in castor oil helps to reduce inflammation and improve blood circulation, which can ease the pain associated with menstrual cramps.

One of the most effective ways to use castor oil for menstrual cramps is through castor oil packs. To make a castor oil pack, soak a piece of flannel cloth in castor oil and place it on the lower abdomen. Cover the cloth with plastic wrap and apply a heating pad or hot water bottle on top to provide gentle heat. The heat helps to enhance the absorption of castor oil through the skin and into the underlying tissues, promoting relaxation and reducing muscle spasms. Leave the pack on for at least 30 minutes to an hour. This method not only alleviates cramps but also promotes a sense of relaxation and comfort.

Regular use of castor oil packs during the menstrual cycle can help to manage cramps effectively and reduce their severity over time. The soothing and anti-inflammatory effects of castor oil provide a natural, holistic approach to managing menstrual pain without the side effects associated with conventional pain medications.

Regulating Menstrual Cycles

In addition to easing menstrual cramps, castor oil can also play a role in regulating menstrual cycles. Irregular menstrual cycles can be caused by various factors, including hormonal imbalances, stress, and underlying health conditions. Castor oil's ability to support hormonal balance and improve circulation can help to promote regular, healthy menstrual cycles.

The use of castor oil packs can be beneficial in regulating menstrual cycles as well. By applying the packs to the lower abdomen, castor oil helps to improve blood flow to the reproductive organs and support their optimal function. This improved circulation can aid in balancing hormones and promoting a more regular menstrual cycle.

Furthermore, castor oil's detoxifying properties can help to cleanse the body of toxins that may disrupt hormonal balance. Regular use of castor oil packs can support liver function, which is crucial for hormone metabolism and detoxification. A healthy liver can effectively process and eliminate excess hormones, helping to maintain a balanced hormonal environment.

To use castor oil for regulating menstrual cycles, apply castor oil packs several times a week, especially in the weeks leading up to the menstrual period.

Consistency is key to achieving the best results. By incorporating castor oil into a regular wellness routine, women can experience more predictable and balanced menstrual cycles.

In conclusion, castor oil offers significant benefits for women's menstrual health. Its anti-inflammatory and analgesic properties make it an effective remedy for easing menstrual cramps, while its ability to improve circulation and support hormonal balance can help to regulate menstrual cycles. By using castor oil packs regularly, women can manage menstrual discomfort naturally and promote overall reproductive health. As we delve deeper into the benefits of castor oil for women's health in this chapter, its role in supporting menstrual health becomes increasingly evident, highlighting its importance in natural health practices.

Pregnancy and Postpartum Care

Using Castor Oil During Pregnancy

Pregnancy is a transformative time for women, accompanied by various physical changes and challenges. While castor oil is known for its numerous health benefits, its use during pregnancy requires caution. Historically, castor oil has been used to induce labor due to its strong laxative effects, which stimulate the intestines and can trigger uterine contractions. However, it is crucial to use castor oil under medical supervision during pregnancy to ensure the safety of both the mother and the baby.

One of the safe and beneficial uses of castor oil during pregnancy is for skin care. As the skin stretches to accommodate the growing baby, many women experience itching, dryness, and the development of stretch marks. Castor oil's rich fatty acids and moisturizing properties can help soothe itching and maintain skin elasticity, reducing the likelihood of stretch marks. Regularly massaging castor oil onto the belly, hips, and thighs can keep the skin hydrated and supple, promoting comfort and skin health throughout the pregnancy.

Another potential benefit of castor oil during pregnancy is its ability to alleviate constipation, a common issue due to hormonal changes and the pressure of the growing uterus on the intestines. If approved by a healthcare provider, a small, carefully monitored dose of castor oil can be used to relieve constipation. However, this should only be done under medical supervision to avoid any risk of premature labor.

It is essential to avoid using castor oil to induce labor without the guidance of a healthcare professional. While some midwives may recommend it in certain cases, unsupervised use can lead to complications such as excessive contractions, dehydration, and fetal distress. Always consult with a healthcare provider before using castor oil for any purpose during pregnancy.

Postpartum Recovery with Castor Oil

After childbirth, a woman's body undergoes significant recovery and healing. Castor oil can play a supportive role in postpartum recovery, helping to address common issues such as perineal pain, hemorrhoids, and stretch marks. Its anti-inflammatory and healing properties make it a valuable addition to postpartum care routines.

For perineal pain and healing, castor oil can be used to create soothing compresses. Soak a clean cloth in warm castor oil and apply it to the perineal area for relief from pain and inflammation. This method can promote healing of any tears or episiotomy wounds, providing comfort during the postpartum recovery period. Additionally, castor oil's antimicrobial properties can help prevent infections in the delicate perineal area.

Hemorrhoids are another common postpartum issue, often resulting from the pressure during labor and delivery. Castor oil's anti-inflammatory properties can provide relief from the discomfort associated with hemorrhoids. Applying a small amount of castor oil to the affected area can reduce swelling and soothe pain, promoting faster healing.

Stretch marks, a common concern during and after pregnancy, can also be addressed with castor oil. The oil's deep moisturizing properties help to improve skin elasticity and reduce the appearance of stretch marks. Regular application of castor oil to areas prone to stretch marks can help fade existing marks and prevent new ones from forming, aiding in skin recovery and overall appearance.

In addition to topical applications, castor oil can support postpartum recovery through castor oil packs. These packs can be applied to the abdomen to promote healing and reduce inflammation. The heat from the pack enhances the absorption of castor oil, allowing its anti-inflammatory and detoxifying properties to benefit the internal tissues. This method can help the body recover more quickly after childbirth by promoting uterine contractions and reducing postpartum bleeding.

Castor oil can also be beneficial for breastfeeding mothers. Its application on dry, cracked nipples can provide relief and promote healing, making breastfeeding more comfortable. However, it is important to wash off any residue before nursing to ensure the baby does not ingest the oil.

In conclusion, castor oil offers a range of benefits for pregnancy and postpartum care when used appropriately and under medical supervision. Its moisturizing, anti-inflammatory, and healing properties can address common issues such as skin discomfort, constipation, perineal pain, hemorrhoids, and stretch marks. By incorporating castor oil into their self-care routines, women can experience enhanced comfort and recovery during and after pregnancy. As we explore the various applications of castor oil for women's health, its role in supporting pregnancy and postpartum recovery becomes increasingly evident, highlighting its value in natural health practices.

Hormonal Balance

Supporting Hormonal Health Naturally

Hormonal balance is crucial for overall well-being, impacting everything from mood and energy levels to reproductive health. Castor oil, with its unique composition and therapeutic properties, can play a significant role in supporting hormonal health naturally. Its ability to promote detoxification, improve circulation, and reduce inflammation makes it a valuable ally in maintaining hormonal balance.

One of the primary ways castor oil supports hormonal health is through its impact on the liver. The liver is essential in metabolizing hormones and removing excess hormones from the body. Castor oil packs, applied to the abdominal area, can enhance liver function by improving circulation and stimulating the detoxification process. This helps to regulate hormone levels, reducing symptoms of hormonal imbalances such as mood swings, fatigue, and irregular menstrual cycles.

Additionally, castor oil's anti-inflammatory properties can help alleviate conditions often associated with hormonal imbalances, such as polycystic ovary syndrome (PCOS) and endometriosis. By reducing inflammation in the reproductive organs, castor oil can help manage pain and other symptoms, promoting overall reproductive health.

Regular use of castor oil packs can also support the lymphatic system, which plays a vital role in maintaining hormonal balance. The lymphatic system helps to transport and eliminate toxins and excess hormones, preventing them from accumulating in the body and disrupting hormonal functions. Improved lymphatic drainage can lead to more stable hormone levels and better overall health.

For those experiencing symptoms of hormonal imbalances, incorporating castor oil into a holistic wellness routine can be beneficial. This natural approach, combined with a balanced diet, regular exercise, and stress management, can significantly enhance hormonal health.

In conclusion, castor oil supports hormonal balance through its detoxifying, anti-inflammatory, and circulatory benefits. By incorporating castor oil packs and topical applications into a regular health regimen, individuals can naturally promote hormonal health and alleviate symptoms associated with hormonal imbalances. This highlights castor oil's importance in natural health practices for maintaining overall well-being.

Chapter 6: Castor Oil in Home Remedies

First Aid Applications

Castor oil's myriad of beneficial properties makes it an invaluable addition to any home first aid kit. Its anti-inflammatory, antimicrobial, and moisturizing qualities lend themselves to a variety of first aid applications, particularly in treating minor cuts, burns, and insect bites and stings. These natural healing properties can offer quick and effective relief, promoting faster recovery and preventing infections.

Treating Minor Cuts and Burns

Minor cuts and burns are common injuries that can benefit significantly from the application of castor oil. Its thick consistency creates a protective barrier over wounds, keeping them moist and preventing them from drying out. This barrier not only shields the wound from external contaminants but also facilitates the healing process by maintaining a hydrated environment, which is essential for tissue repair.

When applied to minor cuts, castor oil's antimicrobial properties help to prevent infection. The oil inhibits the growth of bacteria and fungi, reducing the risk of complications and ensuring that the wound heals cleanly. To use castor oil for treating cuts, clean the wound thoroughly with water and a mild antiseptic. Then, apply a small amount of castor oil directly to the wound and cover it with a sterile bandage. Reapply the oil and change the bandage daily to promote healing and prevent infection.

For minor burns, castor oil provides soothing relief and helps to reduce inflammation and pain. Its anti-inflammatory properties minimize swelling and redness, while its moisturizing effects prevent the skin from becoming overly dry and cracking. To treat a burn, first cool the affected area under running water for several minutes to reduce the heat. Gently pat the area dry with a clean cloth, then apply a generous layer of castor oil. Cover the burn with a non-stick gauze pad and secure it in place. Reapply the oil and change the dressing daily to keep the area clean and moist, promoting faster healing.

Castor Oil for Insect Bites and Stings

Insect bites and stings can cause significant discomfort, including itching, swelling, and pain. Castor oil's anti-inflammatory and soothing properties make it an effective remedy for alleviating these symptoms and promoting faster healing. Its thick consistency also helps to create a barrier that protects the bite or sting from further irritation.

To treat insect bites and stings, apply a small amount of castor oil directly to the affected area. The oil's anti-inflammatory action helps to reduce swelling and redness, while its soothing properties alleviate itching and discomfort. For enhanced relief, you can mix castor oil with a few drops of essential oils known for their soothing effects, such as lavender or tea tree oil. These essential oils have additional anti-inflammatory and antiseptic properties, enhancing the overall effectiveness of the treatment.

Another effective method for treating insect bites and stings is to use a castor oil compress. Soak a clean cloth or cotton pad in castor oil and apply it to the affected area. Secure it with a bandage or adhesive tape and leave it on for several hours or overnight. This method helps to maintain continuous contact with the oil, providing prolonged relief and promoting faster healing.

In addition to treating the immediate symptoms of insect bites and stings, castor oil can also help to prevent secondary infections. Its antimicrobial properties inhibit the growth of bacteria, reducing the risk of infection and ensuring that the bite or sting heals properly. Regular application of castor oil can help to manage the discomfort associated with insect bites and stings, providing a natural and effective remedy for these common injuries.

In conclusion, castor oil is a versatile and effective remedy for various first aid applications, including treating minor cuts, burns, and insect bites and stings. Its anti-inflammatory, antimicrobial, and moisturizing properties make it an essential addition to any home first aid kit. By incorporating castor oil into your first aid routine, you can promote faster healing, prevent infections, and alleviate discomfort naturally. As we explore further into the home remedy applications of castor oil in this chapter, its value in everyday health and wellness becomes increasingly evident, highlighting its importance in natural first aid practices.

Everyday Ailments

Relieving Constipation

Constipation is a common ailment that affects people of all ages, often causing discomfort and disruption to daily life. Castor oil has been used for centuries as a natural laxative to relieve constipation due to its potent properties. The primary active component in castor oil, ricinoleic acid, stimulates the intestines, promoting bowel movements and providing relief from constipation.

When ingested, castor oil is broken down in the small intestine, releasing ricinoleic acid. This acid increases the motility of the intestinal muscles, facilitating the movement of stool through the colon. As a result, castor oil typically produces a bowel movement within two to six hours of ingestion, making it an effective solution for acute constipation.

To use castor oil as a laxative, it is crucial to follow the recommended dosage to avoid potential side effects such as cramping or diarrhea. For adults, the typical dose is one to two tablespoons of castor oil taken on an empty stomach. It can be mixed with a small amount of juice or a flavored drink to mask its strong taste. For children, the dose is significantly lower and should be administered only under the guidance of a healthcare professional.

While castor oil is effective for occasional constipation relief, it is not recommended for long-term use due to its potent laxative effects. Chronic constipation should be addressed with a healthcare provider to identify and treat underlying causes. Nonetheless, for temporary relief, castor oil remains a reliable and natural option.

Alleviating Cold and Flu Symptoms

Cold and flu symptoms, such as congestion, sore throat, and muscle aches, can be alleviated with the help of castor oil's therapeutic properties. Its anti-inflammatory and antimicrobial effects, combined with its ability to improve circulation, make it a valuable remedy for managing the discomfort associated with these common illnesses.

One effective method for using castor oil to alleviate cold and flu symptoms is through chest rubs. When applied to the chest, castor oil penetrates deeply, helping to relieve congestion and improve respiratory function. To create a soothing chest rub, mix castor oil with a few drops of eucalyptus or peppermint essential oil, both of which have decongestant and soothing properties. Gently massage the mixture onto the chest and throat, covering the area with a warm cloth to enhance absorption and provide additional relief.

For sore throats, castor oil can be used as part of a warm compress. Soak a cloth in warm castor oil and apply it to the throat, covering it with a dry towel to retain heat. The warmth and anti-inflammatory properties of castor oil can help reduce throat pain and inflammation, providing comfort and relief.

Castor oil packs can also be beneficial in alleviating muscle aches associated with the flu. Apply a castor oil pack to areas of muscle soreness, such as the back or legs, to reduce inflammation and promote relaxation. The heat from the pack enhances the oil's absorption, providing deeper relief to sore muscles.

Additionally, castor oil can be used to boost the immune system during a cold or flu. Its ability to improve lymphatic circulation helps to enhance the body's natural defenses, supporting faster recovery. Regular application of castor oil packs to the abdomen can stimulate the lymphatic system and improve overall immune function.

In summary, castor oil offers a natural and effective remedy for relieving constipation and alleviating cold and flu symptoms. Its laxative properties provide quick relief from constipation, while its anti-inflammatory and soothing effects help manage the discomfort associated with colds and flu. By incorporating castor oil into your home remedy toolkit, you can address these everyday ailments naturally and effectively. As we delve further into the uses of castor oil for home remedies, its versatility and efficacy in promoting health and wellness become increasingly apparent, highlighting its value in everyday health practices.

Detoxification

Castor Oil Packs

Castor oil packs are a time-honored method of detoxification that utilize the unique properties of castor oil to promote overall health and well-being. These packs involve soaking a piece of flannel cloth in castor oil and applying it to the skin, usually over the liver or abdomen. This method leverages the oil's ability to penetrate deeply into the tissues, enhancing circulation and stimulating the lymphatic system, which is essential for detoxification.

To create a castor oil pack, you will need cold-pressed castor oil, a piece of flannel cloth, plastic wrap, and a heating pad or hot water bottle. Begin by soaking the cloth in castor oil until it is thoroughly saturated. Place the cloth on the desired area, such as the abdomen, and cover it with plastic wrap to prevent the oil from staining clothes or bedding. Apply the heating pad or hot water bottle over the plastic wrap to provide warmth, which helps to enhance the absorption of the oil into the skin. Leave the pack on for about 45 minutes to an hour, allowing the oil to work its way into the tissues and stimulate detoxification processes.

Regular use of castor oil packs can help improve liver function, which plays a crucial role in detoxifying the body. The liver is responsible for filtering toxins from the blood, metabolizing drugs, and processing waste products. By enhancing liver function, castor oil packs support the body's natural detoxification pathways, promoting overall health and vitality. Additionally, the anti-inflammatory properties of castor oil help reduce inflammation in the liver and other organs, further supporting detoxification.

Castor oil packs are also effective in relieving congestion in the lymphatic system. The lymphatic system is responsible for transporting and removing waste products and toxins from the body. By stimulating lymphatic drainage, castor oil packs help to clear these toxins, reducing the burden on the liver and improving overall detoxification. This can lead to increased energy levels, improved digestion, and a strengthened immune system.

Full-Body Detox Methods

Beyond castor oil packs, castor oil can be incorporated into full-body detox methods to support overall detoxification and well-being. One effective approach is to combine castor oil with other detoxifying practices, such as dry brushing, hydrotherapy, and dietary changes.

Dry brushing involves using a natural bristle brush to exfoliate the skin and stimulate lymphatic drainage. Before showering, gently brush your skin in long, sweeping motions towards the heart, focusing on areas where lymph nodes are concentrated, such as the armpits and groin. After dry brushing, apply castor oil to the skin to provide additional hydration and support detoxification.

Hydrotherapy, the use of water for therapeutic purposes, can also be combined with castor oil for detoxification. After a hot bath or sauna session, which helps to open the pores and promote sweating, apply castor oil to the skin to aid in the removal of toxins. The heat from the bath or sauna enhances the absorption of castor oil, allowing it to penetrate deeply and support the detoxification process.

Dietary changes can further enhance the detoxifying effects of castor oil. Incorporate plenty of fresh fruits and vegetables, whole grains, and lean proteins into your diet to support liver function and overall detoxification. Foods rich in antioxidants, such as berries, green tea, and dark leafy greens, help to neutralize free radicals and reduce oxidative stress on the liver. Drinking plenty of water is also essential for flushing out toxins and keeping the body hydrated.

Incorporating castor oil into these full-body detox methods can provide comprehensive support for the body's natural detoxification processes. Regular use of castor oil packs, combined with dry brushing, hydrotherapy, and a healthy diet, can help to eliminate toxins, reduce inflammation, and improve overall health and vitality.

In conclusion, castor oil is a powerful tool for detoxification, offering both targeted and full-body detox methods. Its ability to penetrate deeply into the tissues, stimulate lymphatic drainage, and support liver function makes it an invaluable addition to any detox routine. By incorporating castor oil into your detoxification practices, you can promote overall health and well-being, enhancing the body's natural ability to cleanse and rejuvenate. As we explore further into the home remedy applications of castor oil, its role in detoxification becomes increasingly evident, highlighting its importance in natural health and wellness practices.

Chapter 7: DIY Castor Oil Beauty Recipes

Skin Care Recipes

Castor oil is a versatile and powerful ingredient in many DIY beauty recipes, offering numerous benefits for the skin. Its rich fatty acid content, particularly ricinoleic acid, provides deep hydration, promotes healing, and has anti-inflammatory and antimicrobial properties. Incorporating castor oil into your homemade skin care products can enhance their effectiveness, giving you healthy, radiant skin. In this chapter, we will explore how to create homemade moisturizers, lotions, face masks, and scrubs using castor oil as a key ingredient.

Homemade Moisturizers and Lotions
Creating your own moisturizers and lotions with castor oil can be a rewarding and effective way to tailor skin care products to your specific needs. Castor oil's thick consistency makes it an excellent base for moisturizing formulations, providing long-lasting hydration and protection for the skin.

To make a simple homemade moisturizer, you can combine castor oil with other nourishing oils and butters. Here's a basic recipe:

Ingredients:

2 tablespoons castor oil
2 tablespoons coconut oil
2 tablespoons shea butter
1 tablespoon jojoba oil
5-10 drops of essential oil (optional for fragrance, such as lavender or chamomile)

Instructions:

In a double boiler, melt the coconut oil and shea butter until fully liquefied.

Remove from heat and add the castor oil and jojoba oil. Stir well to combine.

Add the essential oil drops, if using, and mix thoroughly.

Pour the mixture into a clean, sterilized jar and allow it to cool and solidify.

Use this moisturizer daily, applying a small amount to your face and body to keep your skin soft and hydrated.

This simple recipe can be customized by adding other beneficial ingredients like vitamin E oil for its antioxidant properties or aloe vera gel for additional soothing effects.

DIY Face Masks and Scrubs

Face masks and scrubs are essential components of a comprehensive skin care routine, helping to exfoliate, detoxify, and rejuvenate the skin. Castor oil can be effectively incorporated into these DIY treatments to enhance their benefits.

DIY Face Mask Recipe:

Ingredients:

1 tablespoon castor oil

1 tablespoon honey

1 tablespoon plain yogurt

1 teaspoon turmeric powder

Instructions:

In a small bowl, combine all the ingredients and mix until smooth.

Apply the mask evenly to your face, avoiding the eye area.

Leave the mask on for 15-20 minutes.

Rinse off with warm water and gently pat your face dry.

Follow with your regular moisturizer.

This face mask helps to hydrate, brighten, and soothe the skin. Honey and yogurt add moisturizing and exfoliating benefits, while turmeric provides anti-inflammatory and antibacterial properties.

DIY Face Scrub Recipe:

Ingredients:

2 tablespoons castor oil

2 tablespoons finely ground oatmeal

1 tablespoon honey

1 tablespoon lemon juice

Instructions:

In a small bowl, mix all the ingredients until well combined.

Gently massage the scrub onto your damp face in circular motions, focusing on areas that need exfoliation.

Rinse off with warm water and pat your skin dry.

Use this scrub once or twice a week to remove dead skin cells and reveal smoother, brighter skin.

The finely ground oatmeal in this scrub acts as a gentle exfoliant, while honey and lemon juice help to cleanse and brighten the skin. Castor oil ensures that the skin remains hydrated and protected throughout the exfoliation process.

Hair Care Recipes

Castor Oil Shampoos and Conditioners

Creating DIY hair care products using castor oil can transform your hair care routine, providing natural nourishment, promoting hair growth, and improving the overall health of your hair. Castor oil's rich nutrient profile and moisturizing properties make it an excellent ingredient for shampoos and conditioners. These homemade products can help reduce hair loss, add shine, and keep your scalp healthy without the harsh chemicals often found in commercial products.

DIY Castor Oil Shampoo Recipe:

Ingredients:

- 1/4 cup castor oil

- 1/4 cup coconut milk

- 1/4 cup liquid Castile soap

- 10 drops of essential oil (optional, such as lavender or rosemary)

Instructions:

1. In a mixing bowl, combine the castor oil, coconut milk, and liquid Castile soap.

2. Add the essential oil drops if using and stir well to combine.

3. Pour the mixture into a clean, empty shampoo bottle.

4. Shake well before each use. Apply a small amount to your wet hair, massaging it into the scalp and through the ends of your hair.

5. Rinse thoroughly with warm water.

This castor oil shampoo provides gentle cleansing while nourishing the hair and scalp. Coconut milk adds moisture and softness, while liquid Castile soap ensures a thorough cleanse without stripping the hair of its natural oils.

DIY Castor Oil Conditioner Recipe:

Ingredients:

- 2 tablespoons castor oil

- 2 tablespoons aloe vera gel

- 1 tablespoon honey

- 1 tablespoon apple cider vinegar

- 5 drops of essential oil (optional, such as peppermint or tea tree)

Instructions:

1. In a bowl, mix the castor oil, aloe vera gel, honey, and apple cider vinegar until well blended.

2. Add the essential oil drops if using and stir to combine.

3. Apply the mixture to your hair after shampooing, focusing on the ends and any dry areas.

4. Leave the conditioner on for 3-5 minutes before rinsing thoroughly with cool water.

This conditioner deeply hydrates and conditions the hair, leaving it soft, shiny, and manageable. Aloe vera soothes the scalp, honey adds moisture, and apple cider vinegar helps to balance the hair's pH levels and add shine.

Hair Growth Serums

For those looking to boost hair growth and improve hair thickness, castor oil hair growth serums can be an effective and natural solution. Castor oil's high ricinoleic acid content promotes blood circulation to the scalp and nourishes the hair follicles, encouraging healthy hair growth and reducing hair loss.

DIY Hair Growth Serum Recipe:

Ingredients:

- 2 tablespoons castor oil

- 1 tablespoon jojoba oil

- 1 tablespoon argan oil

- 10 drops of rosemary essential oil

- 5 drops of peppermint essential oil

Instructions:

1. In a small bottle with a dropper, combine the castor oil, jojoba oil, and argan oil.

2. Add the rosemary and peppermint essential oils.

3. Shake the bottle well to mix all the ingredients.

4. Apply a few drops of the serum to your scalp, massaging it in gently with your fingertips.

5. Leave the serum on for at least an hour, or overnight for best results, before washing your hair.

This hair growth serum harnesses the power of castor oil and other nourishing oils to stimulate hair growth and improve scalp health. Jojoba oil closely resembles the scalp's natural sebum, making it an excellent moisturizer, while argan oil provides additional nutrients and shine. Rosemary and peppermint essential oils are known for their ability to stimulate hair follicles and promote circulation, enhancing the serum's effectiveness.

DIY Hair Strengthening Serum Recipe:

Ingredients:

- 2 tablespoons castor oil

- 1 tablespoon olive oil

- 1 tablespoon coconut oil

- 10 drops of lavender essential oil

- 5 drops of cedarwood essential oil

Instructions:

1. Combine the castor oil, olive oil, and coconut oil in a small bottle with a dropper.

2. Add the lavender and cedarwood essential oils.

3. Shake the bottle well to blend all the ingredients.

4. Apply a small amount to the scalp and hair, focusing on the roots and ends.

5. Leave the serum on for at least an hour before washing it out with shampoo.

This strengthening serum helps to fortify the hair, reduce breakage, and enhance overall hair health. Olive oil provides deep conditioning, while coconut oil helps to repair damaged hair and prevent protein loss. Lavender and cedarwood essential oils add a soothing aroma and further support hair strength and growth.

In conclusion, incorporating castor oil into your DIY hair care recipes can significantly improve the health, growth, and appearance of your hair. By creating homemade shampoos, conditioners, and hair growth serums, you can enjoy the natural benefits of castor oil while avoiding the harsh chemicals found in many commercial products. As we continue to explore the applications of castor oil in beauty treatments, its versatility and effectiveness in promoting healthy hair become increasingly clear, highlighting its importance in natural hair care practices.

Body Care Recipes

Bath Oils and Body Scrubs

Castor oil is an excellent ingredient for creating luxurious and nourishing body care products. Its rich, emollient properties make it perfect for bath oils and body scrubs that hydrate and exfoliate the skin, leaving it soft and glowing. Incorporating castor oil into your body care routine can transform your bath time into a spa-like experience while providing essential nutrients to your skin.

DIY Bath Oil Recipe:

Ingredients:

- 1/4 cup castor oil

- 1/4 cup sweet almond oil

- 10 drops lavender essential oil

- 5 drops chamomile essential oil

Instructions:

1. In a small bowl, mix the castor oil and sweet almond oil until well blended.

2. Add the lavender and chamomile essential oils and stir to combine.

3. Pour the mixture into a clean, dry bottle with a tight-fitting lid.

4. To use, add a few tablespoons of the bath oil to your running bath water. Swirl the water to distribute the oil evenly.

5. Soak in the bath for at least 20 minutes, allowing the oils to nourish and moisturize your skin.

This bath oil provides deep hydration and relaxation, thanks to the calming scents of lavender and chamomile. Castor oil's thick consistency helps to lock in moisture, while sweet almond oil softens and smooths the skin.

DIY Body Scrub Recipe:

Ingredients:

- 1/2 cup castor oil

- 1/2 cup brown sugar

- 1/4 cup coconut oil (melted)

- 10 drops vanilla essential oil (optional)

Instructions:

1. In a mixing bowl, combine the brown sugar and melted coconut oil.

2. Add the castor oil and vanilla essential oil, stirring until all ingredients are well mixed.

3. Transfer the scrub to a clean, airtight container.

4. In the shower or bath, apply a generous amount of the scrub to your skin, massaging in circular motions to exfoliate.

5. Rinse thoroughly with warm water and pat your skin dry.

This body scrub gently exfoliates dead skin cells while moisturizing the skin. Brown sugar acts as a natural exfoliant, while castor oil and coconut oil provide deep hydration, leaving the skin feeling soft and rejuvenated.

Hand and Foot Treatments

Hands and feet are often neglected in our daily skincare routines, but they require special care to remain soft and healthy. Castor oil can be used to create effective treatments for these areas, addressing issues such as dryness, calluses, and cracked skin.

DIY Hand Treatment Recipe:

Ingredients:

- 2 tablespoons castor oil

- 2 tablespoons shea butter

- 1 tablespoon olive oil

- 5 drops of lavender essential oil

Instructions:

1. In a double boiler, melt the shea butter until fully liquefied.

2. Remove from heat and add the castor oil and olive oil, stirring to combine.

3. Add the lavender essential oil and mix well.

4. Allow the mixture to cool slightly, then pour it into a clean container.

5. Apply a generous amount to your hands before bed, and wear cotton gloves overnight to lock in moisture.

This hand treatment provides intense hydration and healing, especially for dry or chapped hands. The combination of castor oil, shea butter, and olive oil nourishes and repairs the skin, while lavender essential oil adds a soothing aroma.

DIY Foot Treatment Recipe:

Ingredients:

- 2 tablespoons castor oil

- 2 tablespoons coconut oil

- 1 tablespoon beeswax (melted)

- 5 drops peppermint essential oil

Instructions:

1. In a double boiler, melt the beeswax until fully liquefied.

2. Remove from heat and add the castor oil and coconut oil, stirring until well combined.

3. Add the peppermint essential oil and mix thoroughly.

4. Pour the mixture into a clean container and allow it to cool and solidify.

5. Apply the treatment to your feet before bed, focusing on dry or cracked areas, and wear cotton socks overnight.

This foot treatment deeply moisturizes and softens the skin, thanks to the hydrating properties of castor oil and coconut oil. Beeswax helps to seal in moisture, while peppermint essential oil provides a refreshing, cooling sensation.

In conclusion, incorporating castor oil into your body care routine can provide significant benefits for your skin. Whether you are creating bath oils, body scrubs, or hand and foot treatments, castor oil's moisturizing and healing properties make it an invaluable ingredient. These DIY recipes offer natural and effective ways to nourish and pamper your skin, promoting overall health and well-being. As we continue to explore the versatile applications of castor oil in beauty treatments, its role in body care becomes increasingly apparent, highlighting its importance in natural skincare practices.

Chapter 8: Safety and Precautions

Understanding Dosages

While castor oil is a powerful natural remedy with numerous health benefits, it is essential to use it correctly to avoid potential side effects and ensure safety. Understanding the appropriate dosages for different uses and populations is crucial. This chapter focuses on recommended dosages for adults and children, the importance of avoiding overuse, and how to mitigate potential side effects.

Recommended Dosages for Adults and Children

Castor oil's versatility means it can be used both topically and internally, but each method requires careful attention to dosage. When ingested, castor oil acts as a potent laxative, and even small amounts can produce significant effects. Therefore, it is vital to adhere to recommended dosages to prevent adverse reactions.

For adults, the typical oral dosage for relieving constipation is one to two tablespoons (approximately 15 to 30 milliliters). This dose should be taken on an empty stomach, and the effect is usually felt within two to six hours. It is advisable to start with the lower end of the dosage range to assess individual tolerance. Castor oil's strong taste can be mitigated by mixing it with juice or another flavored liquid.

For children over the age of two, the dosage must be significantly lower. A common recommendation is to use one to two teaspoons (approximately 5 to 10 milliliters) for children aged 2 to 12. For children under the age of two, castor oil should only be administered under the guidance of a healthcare professional. As with adults, castor oil should be given on an empty stomach, and its use should be limited to short-term treatment of constipation.

When using castor oil topically, the dosage is less rigid but still important. A small amount of castor oil, typically a few drops to a teaspoon, can be applied directly to the skin or mixed with other oils for broader application. For conditions like arthritis or muscle soreness, applying a generous amount to the affected area and massaging it in can provide relief. For hair and scalp treatments, a few tablespoons can be massaged into the scalp and left on for several hours or overnight.

Avoiding Overuse and Potential Side Effects

While castor oil is generally safe when used appropriately, overuse can lead to unwanted side effects. Internally, excessive consumption of castor oil can cause severe diarrhea, abdominal cramping, dehydration, and electrolyte imbalances. These effects are due to the oil's strong laxative action, which can lead to rapid fluid loss. Therefore, it is crucial not to exceed the recommended dosage and to use castor oil as a laxative only for short periods.

Chronic use of castor oil for constipation is not recommended, as it can lead to dependency and decreased bowel function over time. If constipation persists, it is important to seek medical advice to address the underlying causes rather than relying on frequent use of castor oil.

Topical use of castor oil generally has fewer side effects, but some individuals may experience skin irritation or allergic reactions. It is advisable to perform a patch test before applying castor oil extensively. Apply a small amount to a patch of skin and wait 24 hours to check for any adverse reactions. If redness, itching, or irritation occurs, discontinue use.

Pregnant and breastfeeding women should exercise caution with castor oil. While it has been traditionally used to induce labor, its use should be strictly supervised by a healthcare provider due to the risk of strong uterine contractions and potential complications. Breastfeeding women should also consult with a healthcare professional before using castor oil, especially when considering internal use.

In conclusion, understanding the appropriate dosages and potential side effects of castor oil is essential for safe and effective use. By adhering to recommended dosages and being mindful of the risks of overuse, individuals can enjoy the numerous benefits of castor oil while minimizing the likelihood of adverse effects. As we continue to explore the various applications of castor oil, maintaining safety and precaution remains paramount to harnessing its full potential in health and wellness practices.

Interactions and Contraindications

Safe Use with Medications

While castor oil is generally safe for many people when used appropriately, it is important to be aware of potential interactions with medications and certain health conditions. Understanding these interactions and contraindications can help ensure that castor oil is used safely and effectively.

Castor oil can interact with certain medications, particularly those that affect the gastrointestinal system. For example, using castor oil as a laxative can interfere with the absorption of other oral medications, reducing their effectiveness. It is advisable to take castor oil and other medications at different times, allowing a few hours in between to ensure proper absorption.

Patients taking medications for chronic conditions such as heart disease, diabetes, or high blood pressure should consult their healthcare provider before using castor oil, especially if considering internal use. Castor oil's laxative effect can lead to dehydration and electrolyte imbalances, which could exacerbate these conditions or interfere with the effectiveness of prescribed medications.

People taking blood thinners or anticoagulant medications should exercise caution with castor oil. While castor oil is not known to have significant anticoagulant properties, any potential interactions with blood thinners should be discussed with a healthcare provider to avoid complications.

For individuals on immunosuppressive medications or those with compromised immune systems, it is important to consider the potential impact of castor oil on immune function. While topical use is generally safe, internal use should be monitored closely to prevent adverse effects on immune health.

Who Should Avoid Castor Oil

Certain individuals should avoid using castor oil due to potential health risks and contraindications. Pregnant women, as mentioned earlier, should be particularly cautious. Although castor oil has been used historically to induce labor, it can cause strong uterine contractions and potentially lead to premature labor or other complications. Therefore, its use during pregnancy should only be under the guidance of a healthcare provider.

Breastfeeding mothers should also be cautious. While topical use of castor oil is generally considered safe, internal use may affect the infant through breast milk. It is best to consult with a healthcare provider before using castor oil internally while breastfeeding.

Individuals with gastrointestinal disorders such as irritable bowel syndrome (IBS), Crohn's disease, or ulcerative colitis should avoid using castor oil as a laxative. Its strong purgative effects can aggravate these conditions, leading to severe cramping, diarrhea, and dehydration. Those with gastrointestinal conditions should seek alternative, milder remedies for constipation and digestive issues.

People with a known allergy to castor oil or its components should obviously avoid using it. Symptoms of an allergic reaction can include itching, swelling, rash, and difficulty breathing. If any of these symptoms occur after using castor oil, discontinue use immediately and seek medical attention.

Patients with kidney disease should also exercise caution when using castor oil internally. The laxative effect of castor oil can lead to significant fluid loss, which can strain the kidneys and worsen kidney function. It is crucial for individuals with kidney issues to consult their healthcare provider before using castor oil as a laxative.

Individuals with certain chronic health conditions, such as heart disease or electrolyte imbalances, should be cautious with castor oil use. The potential for dehydration and electrolyte disturbances from its laxative effect can pose significant risks. Healthcare providers can offer guidance on whether castor oil is appropriate and safe for these individuals.

In conclusion, while castor oil offers numerous health benefits, it is essential to understand its interactions and contraindications to ensure safe use. Being aware of potential interactions with medications and recognizing who should avoid castor oil can help prevent adverse effects and enhance the overall safety of its application. By consulting with healthcare providers and using castor oil mindfully, individuals can safely incorporate this natural remedy into their health and wellness routines. As we continue to explore the various applications of castor oil, maintaining an informed and cautious approach is key to harnessing its full potential while safeguarding health.

Purchasing and Storing Castor Oil

Selecting High-Quality Castor Oil

To fully benefit from castor oil's therapeutic properties, it is essential to select high-quality oil. Not all castor oils are created equal, and the quality can significantly impact its effectiveness and safety. Here are key factors to consider when purchasing castor oil:

1. Cold-Pressed and Hexane-Free: Look for castor oil that is cold-pressed and hexane-free. Cold-pressing ensures that the oil is extracted without the use of heat, preserving its natural nutrients and beneficial compounds. Hexane-free means that no harmful chemicals were used in the extraction process, making the oil safer for use.

2. Organic Certification: Choosing organic castor oil ensures that the oil is free from pesticides, synthetic fertilizers, and other harmful chemicals. Organic certification guarantees that the castor beans were grown under stringent organic farming standards, providing a purer and more natural product.

3. Purity and Additives: High-quality castor oil should be 100% pure and free from additives, fillers, and artificial ingredients. Always check the ingredient list to ensure that you are getting pure castor oil without any unnecessary additives that could dilute its potency or cause adverse reactions.

4. Color and Viscosity: Pure castor oil typically has a pale yellow color and a thick, viscous consistency. Be cautious of oils that are very light or have an unusual color, as this could indicate that the oil has been refined or mixed with other substances.

5. Packaging: The packaging of castor oil is also an important consideration. Dark glass bottles are ideal because they protect the oil from light, which can degrade its quality over time. Avoid oils packaged in clear plastic bottles, as they offer less protection against light and may contain harmful chemicals.

By selecting high-quality castor oil, you can ensure that you are getting a product that is both safe and effective, allowing you to fully enjoy its health and beauty benefits.

Proper Storage Techniques

Proper storage of castor oil is essential to maintain its quality and extend its shelf life. Here are some tips on how to store castor oil correctly:

1. Keep It Cool and Dark: Store castor oil in a cool, dark place, away from direct sunlight and heat sources. Light and heat can cause the oil to degrade, reducing its effectiveness and shelf life. A pantry or a cupboard away from the stove or other heat-producing appliances is an ideal storage location.

2. Use Dark Glass Containers: If your castor oil did not come in a dark glass bottle, consider transferring it to one. Dark glass containers help protect the oil from light exposure, which can cause oxidation and spoilage. Ensure the container is clean and dry before transferring the oil.

3. Seal Tightly: Always keep the bottle tightly sealed when not in use. Exposure to air can cause the oil to oxidize and go rancid over time. A tightly sealed bottle will help preserve the oil's freshness and potency.

4. Avoid Contamination: To prevent contamination, avoid dipping your fingers or unclean utensils directly into the bottle. Instead, pour a small amount of oil into a separate, clean container for use. This practice helps maintain the purity of the remaining oil in the bottle.

5. Monitor Shelf Life: While castor oil has a relatively long shelf life, typically up to a year, it's essential to check for signs of spoilage periodically. If the oil develops an off smell, changes color, or has a different consistency, it may have gone rancid and should be discarded.

6. Refrigeration (Optional): Although not necessary, storing castor oil in the refrigerator can extend its shelf life, especially if you live in a warm climate. However, keep in mind that refrigeration may cause the oil to thicken. If this happens, simply bring it to room temperature before use.

By following these proper storage techniques, you can ensure that your castor oil remains fresh, potent, and effective for an extended period. Properly stored castor oil will retain its beneficial properties, allowing you to make the most of this versatile natural remedy.

In conclusion, selecting high-quality castor oil and storing it correctly are crucial steps in ensuring its efficacy and safety. By choosing cold-pressed, organic, and pure castor oil, and by protecting it from light, heat, and air, you can maintain its therapeutic properties and enjoy its full range of health and beauty benefits. As we continue to explore the various applications of castor oil, understanding how to purchase and store it properly becomes increasingly important, highlighting its role in natural health and wellness practices.

Chapter 9: Sourcing and Sustainability

Ethical Sourcing

As awareness of environmental and social issues grows, ethical sourcing has become a crucial aspect of purchasing castor oil. Ethical sourcing ensures that the production and procurement of castor oil do not harm the environment, exploit workers, or contribute to unsustainable agricultural practices. By understanding how castor oil is produced and identifying ethical suppliers, consumers can make informed choices that support sustainability and fair trade.

How Castor Oil is Produced

Castor oil is derived from the seeds of the Ricinus communis plant, commonly known as the castor bean plant. The production process involves several stages, from cultivation and harvesting to extraction and refinement. Understanding this process can help highlight the importance of sustainable practices at each stage.

1. **Cultivation and Harvesting**: The castor bean plant thrives in tropical and subtropical regions. It requires specific climatic conditions, including warm temperatures and well-drained soil. Ethical sourcing begins with sustainable farming practices that minimize environmental impact. This includes using organic farming methods, avoiding synthetic fertilizers and pesticides, and implementing crop rotation to maintain soil health.

2. **Extraction**: The extraction process typically involves cold pressing the castor beans to obtain the oil. Cold pressing is a mechanical method that does not involve heat or chemicals, preserving the oil's natural properties and nutrients. This method is not only beneficial for maintaining the oil's

quality but also for reducing environmental pollution and energy consumption compared to chemical extraction processes.

3. **Refinement**: After extraction, the oil may undergo refinement to remove impurities. Ethical refining processes avoid harmful chemicals and focus on maintaining the oil's purity and potency. Some suppliers may offer unrefined castor oil, which retains more of its natural nutrients and is preferred for its holistic benefits.

4. **Packaging and Distribution**: Sustainable packaging and distribution practices further contribute to the overall ethical sourcing of castor oil. This includes using recyclable or biodegradable packaging materials and implementing efficient distribution methods to reduce carbon footprints.

Identifying Ethical Suppliers

Identifying ethical suppliers of castor oil involves looking for specific certifications and practices that ensure the product is sourced responsibly. Here are some key factors to consider:

1. **Certifications**: Look for certifications such as USDA Organic, Fair Trade, and EcoCert. These certifications indicate that the product meets stringent standards for organic farming, fair labor practices, and environmental sustainability. Certified organic castor oil ensures that the product is free from synthetic chemicals and is produced using sustainable agricultural methods.

2. **Fair Trade Practices**: Suppliers that adhere to fair trade principles ensure that farmers and workers are paid fair wages, work in safe conditions, and have access to necessary resources. Fair trade certification also promotes community development and environmental stewardship.

3. **Sustainable Farming Practices**: Ethical suppliers prioritize sustainable farming practices that protect the environment and promote biodiversity. This includes using organic farming methods, conserving water, and protecting natural habitats. Suppliers committed to sustainability often provide detailed information about their farming practices and the steps they take to minimize environmental impact.

4. **Transparent Supply Chain**: Ethical suppliers maintain transparency in their supply chain, providing information about the origins of their products and the methods used in production. Transparency builds trust with consumers and ensures that the product is sourced responsibly.

5. **Community and Environmental Impact**: Consider suppliers that actively contribute to the well-being of the communities where castor oil is produced. This can include initiatives such as supporting local education, healthcare, and infrastructure projects, as well as efforts to reduce environmental impact through reforestation and conservation programs.

By prioritizing ethical sourcing, consumers can support sustainable practices that benefit both people and the planet. Choosing castor oil from ethical suppliers ensures that the product is not only of high quality but also produced in a way that respects the environment and promotes social justice.

In conclusion, understanding how castor oil is produced and identifying ethical suppliers are essential steps in ensuring that the product you purchase aligns with your values of sustainability and fairness. By supporting ethical sourcing, consumers can contribute to a more sustainable and equitable world, making a positive impact on both the environment and the communities involved in castor oil production. As we continue to explore the benefits and applications of castor oil, recognizing the importance of ethical sourcing becomes increasingly important, highlighting its role in promoting global sustainability and social responsibility.

Environmental Impact

The Environmental Benefits of Castor Oil

Castor oil production offers several environmental benefits, contributing positively to sustainable agriculture and the reduction of ecological footprints. The castor bean plant, Ricinus communis, is a resilient and adaptable crop that can thrive in a variety of climates and soil types, often requiring fewer resources compared to other commercial crops.

1. **Drought Resistance**: One of the significant environmental benefits of the castor bean plant is its drought resistance. The plant can grow in arid and semi-arid regions with minimal water requirements, reducing the strain on water resources. This makes it a viable crop in areas that are unsuitable for other types of agriculture, promoting the use of otherwise underutilized land.

2. **Low Input Requirements**: Castor plants typically require fewer chemical inputs such as fertilizers and pesticides compared to other commercial crops. This not only reduces the risk of soil and water contamination but also lowers the overall environmental impact of its cultivation. Organic farming practices further enhance these benefits by eliminating synthetic inputs altogether.

3. **Soil Health**: The castor bean plant has deep root systems that help improve soil structure and prevent erosion. These roots can enhance soil fertility by breaking up compacted soil layers and increasing water infiltration.

Additionally, castor plants can be integrated into crop rotation systems, contributing to sustainable farming practices that maintain and improve soil health.

4. **Carbon Sequestration**: Like other plants, castor bean plants absorb carbon dioxide during photosynthesis, helping to mitigate the effects of climate change. By sequestering carbon, castor cultivation can contribute to reducing the overall carbon footprint of agricultural activities.

5. **Biodegradability**: Castor oil is a biodegradable substance, meaning it breaks down naturally without causing environmental harm. This makes it an eco-friendly alternative to synthetic oils and chemicals, which can persist in the environment and contribute to pollution.

6. **Renewable Resource**: Castor oil is derived from a renewable resource – the seeds of the castor bean plant. Unlike fossil fuels and other non-renewable resources, castor oil production is sustainable over the long term, provided that ethical and environmentally friendly farming practices are maintained.

Reducing Your Ecological Footprint

Consumers can play a crucial role in reducing their ecological footprint by choosing products made from castor oil and incorporating sustainable practices into their daily lives. Here are several ways to do so:

1. **Choose Sustainable Products**: Opt for products that use castor oil as a primary ingredient, such as biodegradable plastics, eco-friendly lubricants, and natural cosmetics. By selecting these products, you support industries that prioritize sustainable raw materials and reduce reliance on petroleum-based products.

2. **Support Ethical Brands**: Purchase castor oil and castor oil-based products from brands that demonstrate a commitment to environmental sustainability and ethical sourcing. Look for certifications and transparency in their production processes to ensure your purchase supports environmentally responsible practices.

3. **DIY Solutions**: Create your own beauty and household products using castor oil. This not only reduces the consumption of products with synthetic ingredients and excessive packaging but also allows you to control the quality and sustainability of the ingredients used. Recipes for homemade moisturizers, shampoos, and cleaning agents often include castor oil as a key ingredient due to its versatility and effectiveness.

4. **Reduce Plastic Use**: Many conventional products come in plastic packaging that contributes to environmental pollution. By choosing castor oil-based products, which are often packaged in recyclable or biodegradable materials, you can help reduce plastic waste. Additionally, consider purchasing castor oil in bulk to minimize packaging waste.

5. **Educate and Advocate**: Raise awareness about the environmental benefits of castor oil and encourage others to make sustainable choices. Advocacy and education can drive demand for eco-friendly products and support the growth of sustainable industries.

6. **Sustainable Farming Practices**: If you are involved in agriculture or gardening, consider growing castor bean plants using sustainable practices. This can contribute to local biodiversity, improve soil health, and reduce the need for chemical inputs. Sharing knowledge and techniques with other growers can help expand the positive environmental impact.

7. **Reduce Chemical Use**: Replace chemical-based products in your home with castor oil alternatives. For example, use castor oil-based soaps and detergents, which are biodegradable and less harmful to aquatic ecosystems compared to conventional products.

In conclusion, castor oil production and use offer significant environmental benefits, contributing to sustainable agriculture and reducing ecological footprints. By choosing products made from castor oil and supporting ethical and environmentally responsible brands, consumers can help promote sustainability and reduce environmental impact. As we explore the various applications of castor oil, its role in promoting environmental health becomes increasingly clear, underscoring its importance in the pursuit of a more sustainable and eco-friendly future.

Homemade Castor Oil Production

Making Castor Oil at Home

Producing castor oil at home can be a rewarding and educational experience, providing you with a pure and high-quality product. While the process requires some time and effort, it allows for complete control over the ingredients and methods used, ensuring that the final product is free from additives and contaminants. Here is a step-by-step guide to making castor oil at home:

1. **Harvesting and Preparing Castor Beans**: The first step in making castor oil at home is to obtain high-quality castor beans. If you have access to a castor bean plant, you can harvest the seeds when they are fully mature and dry. Be sure to handle the seeds with care, as they contain ricin, a toxic compound. Always wear gloves and work in a well-ventilated area to avoid exposure.

2. **Cleaning the Seeds**: Thoroughly clean the harvested seeds to remove any dirt or debris. Rinse them under running water and let them dry completely.

3. **Heating the Seeds**: To facilitate oil extraction, lightly roast the seeds in a pan over low heat. This step helps to break down the seeds' structure, making it easier to extract the oil. Be cautious not to burn the seeds, as this can affect the oil's quality.

4. **Grinding the Seeds**: Once the seeds are roasted, grind them into a coarse powder using a grinder or mortar and pestle. This step increases the surface area, making oil extraction more efficient.

5. **Pressing the Oil**: The most common method for extracting oil is cold pressing. You can use a manual or electric oil press to extract the oil from the ground seeds. If you don't have access to an oil press, you can place the ground seeds in a cloth bag and apply pressure using a heavy object or a homemade press.

6. **Filtering the Oil**: After pressing, the extracted oil may contain impurities and seed particles. Filter the oil through a fine mesh strainer or cheesecloth to remove these impurities. For a clearer product, you can repeat this filtering process several times.

7. **Storing the Oil**: Transfer the filtered oil into a clean, dark glass bottle with a tight-fitting lid. Store the bottle in a cool, dark place to protect the oil from light and heat, which can degrade its quality over time.

Ensuring Purity and Quality

Ensuring the purity and quality of homemade castor oil requires attention to detail and adherence to best practices throughout the production process. Here are some tips to help you produce the highest quality castor oil at home:

1. **Use Fresh, High-Quality Seeds**: The quality of the castor beans significantly impacts the final product. Use fresh, high-quality seeds from a reliable source. Avoid using old or spoiled seeds, as they can produce rancid or low-quality oil.

2. **Maintain Cleanliness**: Cleanliness is crucial when producing castor oil at home. Ensure that all equipment, utensils, and containers are thoroughly cleaned and sterilized before use. This helps prevent contamination and ensures the purity of the oil.

3. **Proper Roasting**: Roast the seeds lightly to aid in oil extraction without burning them. Over-roasting can alter the oil's properties and reduce its effectiveness.

4. **Efficient Grinding**: Grind the seeds thoroughly to increase the efficiency of oil extraction. The finer the grind, the more oil you can extract from the seeds.

5. **Cold Pressing Method**: Cold pressing is the preferred method for extracting castor oil, as it preserves the oil's natural properties and nutrients.

Avoid using heat-based extraction methods, which can degrade the oil's quality.

6. **Thorough Filtering**: Filter the oil multiple times to remove any remaining impurities and seed particles. This ensures that the final product is clear and pure, suitable for various applications.

7. **Proper Storage**: Store the oil in a dark glass bottle to protect it from light and air exposure, which can cause oxidation and spoilage. Keep the bottle tightly sealed and store it in a cool, dark place to maintain the oil's freshness and potency.

8. **Labeling and Dating**: Label the bottle with the production date to keep track of its shelf life. While properly stored castor oil can last up to a year, it is best to use it within six months for optimal freshness and effectiveness.

By following these steps and tips, you can produce high-quality castor oil at home, ensuring its purity and effectiveness for various health and beauty applications. Homemade castor oil not only provides a cost-effective alternative to store-bought options but also offers the satisfaction of creating a natural product with complete control over the ingredients and process.

In conclusion, making castor oil at home is a rewarding endeavor that allows for the production of pure, high-quality oil. By harvesting, preparing, and processing the seeds carefully, you can ensure that your homemade castor oil is free from additives and contaminants. Proper storage techniques further guarantee the oil's freshness and potency, making it a valuable addition to your natural health and beauty regimen. As we explore the various applications of castor oil, understanding how to produce and maintain its quality at home highlights its versatility and importance in natural wellness practices.

Chapter 10: Testimonials and Case Studies

Real-Life Success Stories

Castor oil's remarkable benefits have been experienced and shared by countless individuals, highlighting its versatility and effectiveness in promoting health and beauty. These real-life success stories and case studies provide compelling evidence of castor oil's transformative effects.

Health Transformations with Castor Oil

Many people have found relief from chronic conditions and significant health improvements by incorporating castor oil into their wellness routines. For instance, individuals suffering from arthritis have reported reduced pain and increased mobility after regularly using castor oil packs. Similarly, those with digestive issues have experienced relief from constipation and improved digestive health through the careful use of castor oil as a natural laxative.

Beauty Enhancements Through Natural Remedies

Castor oil has also been celebrated for its ability to enhance beauty naturally. Users have shared stories of improved hair growth, thickness, and shine by using castor oil-based hair treatments. In skincare, individuals have noticed clearer, more hydrated skin and a reduction in acne and blemishes. These testimonials underscore castor oil's efficacy as a natural alternative to conventional beauty products, providing both health and aesthetic benefits.

These success stories and case studies serve as powerful testimonials to the efficacy of castor oil, inspiring others to explore its potential for improving health and beauty naturally. As we delve deeper into these narratives, the transformative impact of castor oil on real lives becomes undeniably clear.

Expert Opinions

Insights from Health and Wellness Experts

Health and wellness experts frequently endorse castor oil for its wide-ranging benefits. Nutritionists and naturopaths often recommend castor oil for its anti-inflammatory and detoxifying properties, advocating its use in natural health regimens. Experts emphasize castor oil's role in promoting digestive health, relieving constipation, and supporting liver detoxification. Additionally, holistic health practitioners highlight its efficacy in enhancing skin and hair care, citing its deep moisturizing and healing effects.

Medical Perspectives on Castor Oil Use

Medical professionals also acknowledge the therapeutic potential of castor oil, particularly in its use as a natural remedy for various conditions. Dermatologists recognize its benefits in treating skin ailments such as acne, eczema, and psoriasis due to its antimicrobial and anti-inflammatory properties. Rheumatologists sometimes recommend castor oil packs for patients with arthritis to alleviate joint pain and inflammation. Gastroenterologists may suggest its cautious use as a laxative for short-term relief of constipation.

These expert insights and medical perspectives reinforce the value of castor oil as a versatile, natural remedy. By integrating expert opinions, this chapter underscores the scientific and practical support for castor oil's diverse applications in health and wellness, providing a balanced view of its benefits and recommended uses.

Your Journey with Castor Oil

Tracking Your Progress

Embarking on your journey with castor oil involves more than just integrating it into your daily routine; it also requires mindful tracking of your progress. Keeping a journal to document your experiences can be incredibly beneficial. Note any improvements in health conditions, changes in skin and hair texture, or relief from symptoms. By tracking the frequency and methods of castor oil use, you can identify what works best for you and make informed adjustments as needed. This systematic approach helps in understanding the full extent of castor oil's benefits and optimizing its use for your personal needs.

Sharing Your Story

Sharing your castor oil journey can inspire and inform others who might benefit from its diverse applications. Whether through social media, blog posts, or community forums, discussing your experiences can provide valuable insights and encouragement to others exploring natural remedies. Your success stories and practical tips on using castor oil for health and beauty can help build a supportive community of users who share a common interest in natural wellness. By contributing your voice, you not only celebrate your achievements but also help spread awareness of castor oil's potential, fostering a collective journey toward better health and well-being.

Conclusion

Bringing It All Together

Throughout this guide, we've explored the myriad benefits of castor oil, from its historical uses to modern applications in health, beauty, and wellness. Its versatility and effectiveness make it a valuable addition to any natural health regimen. By understanding how to use castor oil safely and effectively, you can harness its full potential to enhance your well-being.

Integrating Castor Oil into Your Daily Life

Incorporating castor oil into your daily routine is straightforward and can yield significant results. Whether you use it for skin care, hair treatments, or as a remedy for digestive and menstrual issues, consistency is key. Simple applications, such as adding it to your moisturizers, creating hair masks, or using castor oil packs, can make a noticeable difference in your health and appearance.

Long-Term Benefits and Continued Use

The long-term benefits of castor oil are profound. Regular use can lead to sustained improvements in skin hydration, hair strength, and overall health. Its natural properties promote healing, reduce inflammation, and support bodily functions. By continuing to use castor oil as part of a holistic approach to wellness, you can enjoy its benefits for years to come.

In conclusion, castor oil is a powerful, natural ally in maintaining and improving your health. As you integrate it into your daily life, you will likely discover even more ways it can support your journey towards better health and wellness. Embrace the journey and let castor oil be a cornerstone of your natural health regimen.

Resources and Further Reading

Additional Books and Articles

Expanding your knowledge about castor oil and its applications can be immensely beneficial. Consider exploring books such as "The Miracle of Castor Oil" by JJ Stanley, which delves into the science and history of castor oil use. Another valuable resource is "Castor Oil: The Natural Remedy Guide" by John Davidson, offering detailed insights and practical tips. Additionally, scientific journals and articles on natural health and wellness can provide in-depth information on the benefits and mechanisms of castor oil.

Helpful Websites and Blogs

Several websites and blogs are dedicated to natural health and the use of castor oil. Websites like Wellness Mama and Dr. Axe offer articles, recipes, and user testimonials on incorporating castor oil into daily routines. The National Center for Biotechnology Information (NCBI) provides access to research studies and scientific data on the health benefits of castor oil. Blogs such as The Healthy Home Economist and The Natural Haven Bloom also offer practical tips, personal experiences, and expert advice on using castor oil for health and beauty purposes.

Made in United States
Orlando, FL
31 May 2025

61727382R00050